New Horizons of Exercise Medicine

Edited by Hidetaka Hamasaki

Published in London, United Kingdom

New Horizons of Exercise Medicine
http://dx.doi.org/10.5772/intechopen.1002112
Edited by Hidetaka Hamasaki

Contributors
Alberto Romano, Dae Taek Lee, Dimitra Koutsouki, Endang Ernandini, Hajer Alhinai, Hidetaka Hamasaki, İlkim Çıtak Karakaya, Jonathan Alvin Wiryaputra, Katerina Asonitou, Leo Bockeria, Meir Lotan, Musa Çankaya, Nona Pachuashvili, Shan Gao, Soteria Yiannaki, Tamara Dzhitava, Tea Kakuchaya, Yongsuk Seo, Zarina Tokaeva, Zuowei Pei

First published in London, United Kingdom, 2024 by IntechOpen
IntechOpen is the global imprint of INTECHOPEN LIMITED, registered in England and Wales, registration number: 11086078, 167-169 Great Portland Street, London, W1W 5PF, United Kingdom

British Library Cataloguing-in-Publication Data
A catalogue record for this book is available from the British Library

Additional hard and PDF copies can be obtained from orders@intechopen.com

New Horizons of Exercise Medicine
Edited by Hidetaka Hamasaki
p. cm.
Print ISBN 978-0-85466-608-9
Online ISBN 978-0-85466-607-2
eBook (PDF) ISBN 978-0-85466-609-6

Meet the editor

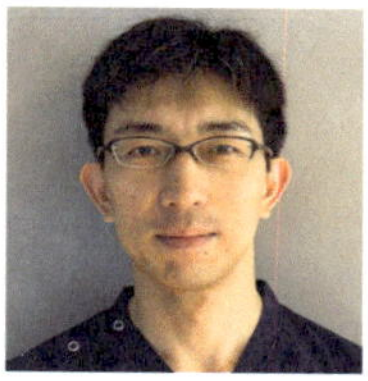

Dr. Hidetaka Hamasaki serves as the director of the Hamasaki Clinic. His primary areas of interest include diabetes, endocrinology, physical activity, and exercise medicine. Dr. Hamasaki is a prolific author, having contributed to more than 100 scientific papers on exercise medicine, especially the relationship between metabolic disorders and physical activity in diabetes patients, as well as the association between handgrip strength and cardiovascular diseases. He is an esteemed member of several professional societies, such as the American College of Physicians, the Japanese Society of Internal Medicine, the Japan Diabetes Society, the Japanese Society of Physical Fitness and Sports Medicine, and SigmaXi. He also serves as an academic editor in several scientific journals including PLOS ONE.

Contents

Preface

Welcome to *New Horizons of Exercise Medicine*, a comprehensive guide to understanding the role of exercise in promoting health and well-being. This book explores the latest research, practical strategies, and insights into how exercise can be used as medicine to prevent and manage various health conditions.

Our goal is to provide readers with a deep understanding of the physiological, psychological, and social benefits of exercise. Whether you are a healthcare professional, fitness enthusiast, or someone looking to improve their health, this book offers valuable information and tools to support your journey toward a healthier lifestyle.

In the first section, after the introductory chapter, Dr. Katerina Asonitou and colleagues delve into the historical utilization of exercise for medical purposes, providing a comprehensive overview of the scientific evidence in their chapter titled "Exercise Is Medicine through Time: Prescription of Adapted Physical Activity in Treatment and Rehabilitation". They also address the promotion of physical activity for health benefits and societal barriers to exercise medicine. Dr. Endang Ernandini and Dr. Jonathan Alvin Wiryaputra further explore the physiological impacts of exercise on humans and its comprehensive health benefits in their chapter titled "Exercise is Medicine".

Moving on to the second section, the book discusses the effects of exercise on various health conditions such as dyslipidemia, coronary artery disease, and cancers. Dr. Xueqi Lin and Dr. Zuowei Pei present a brief overview of the main pathogenic factors of hyperlipidemia in daily life, followed by a detailed discussion on the impact and effectiveness of lifestyle intervention on hyperlipidemia in their chapter titled "Effect and Improvement of Lifestyle Intervention on Hyperlipidemia". Additionally in chapter "A New Algorithm for the Selection and Risk Stratification of Patients for the Efficient Aerobic Cardiorespiratory Training after Coronary Artery Bypass Surgery", Dr. Tea Kakuchaya and colleagues introduce a novel risk stratification algorithm for exercise medicine in post-coronary artery bypass surgery patients based on their clinical study findings. Dr. Hajer Alhinai summarizes the evidence regarding the effectiveness of exercises on clinical symptoms related to the treatment of cancer patients in the chapter titled "Supportive Exercises For Cancer Patients". This chapter presents brief evidence of the effects of exercises on the side effects associated with cancer treatments, including cancer-related fatigue, lymphedema, chemotherapy-induced peripheral neuropathy, urinary incontinence, osteoporosis, and cachexia.

In the third section, the book introduces new and specific exercise modalities. Dr. Yongsuk Seo and Dr. Dae Taek Lee discuss the effectiveness of Self-Natural Posture Exercise in individuals with chronic pain and musculoskeletal conditions in their chapter "A Healthy Life with Self-Natural Posture Exercise". Dr. Musa Çankaya and Dr. İlkim Çıtak Karakaya highlight the strengths of isokinetic exercises, particularly Russian and Aussie currents, which are beneficial for treating various diseases as part of exercise therapy in their chapter "Using Burst Modality Medium Frequency Alternating (Russian and Aussie) Currents with Isokinetic Training". Finally, in the chapter "Health Promotion Through Advanced Physical Activity Programs for Individuals with Intellectual and Developmental Disabilities", Dr. Meir Lotan and Dr. Alberto Romano provide a comprehensive summary of information and evidence on Intellectual and Developmental Disabilities, emphasizing the usefulness of exercise therapy for this condition.

I would like to express our gratitude to all the experts and researchers whose work has contributed to the knowledge shared in this book.

I hope that *New Horizons of Exercise Medicine* will inspire you to embrace the power of exercise and integrate it into your daily life for optimal health and vitality.

Best wishes,

Hidetaka Hamasaki
Hamasaki Clinic,
Kagoshima, Japan

Section 1

What is Exercise Medicine

Chapter 1

Introductory Chapter: Exercise Medicine – Past, Present, and Future

Hidetaka Hamasaki

1. Introduction

1.1 Exercise is medicine

In 1907, Dr. Theodore Toepel lamented that very few physicians possessed the necessary skills and knowledge to recommend "physical exercise" as a therapeutic method for diseases, understanding its effects and limits [1]. More than a century has passed since then, and exercise is now widely recognized as a reliable, validated, and effective form of medicine for patients with various conditions. Surprisingly, a PubMed search using the term "exercise medicine" yielded over 180,000 articles as of October 22, 2023, and the scientific evidence in this field continues to grow.

The "Exercise is Medicine" initiative began in the 1990s, based on a significant study published in 1989 that revealed a clear link between low physical fitness levels and an increased risk of all-cause mortality, including cardiovascular diseases and cancers [2]. In 2007, the American Medical Association and the American College of Sports Medicine jointly introduced the health initiative "Exercise is MedicineTM," emphasizing that "if we had a pill that could confer all the proven health benefits of exercise, physicians would readily prescribe it to their patients, and our healthcare system would ensure that every patient had access to this wonder drug" [3].

Currently, exercise medicine is integrated into daily clinical practice for patients dealing with noncommunicable diseases, such as diabetes and cancer, and for those undergoing rehabilitation as a standard procedure. Furthermore, exercise not only ameliorates disease conditions but also helps prevent the development of certain chronic diseases. For example, exercise reduces the risk of cardiovascular diseases by improving autonomic balance and inducing a cardioprotective effect, through the release of anti-inflammatory cytokines, stimulation of myocardial regeneration, and enhancement of muscle strength and mass [4]. Substantial evidence suggests that exercise effectively reduces the risk of various cancers, including breast, colon, uterine, esophageal, stomach, and renal cancers, through physiological and biochemical changes, such as regulating cell growth, repairing DNA damage, modulating epigenetic expression, regulating apoptosis, harmonizing endocrine functions (e.g. myokines and sex hormones), improving immune function, and reducing oxidative stress and inflammation [5]. Recently, exercise has also been proposed as a potential means of reducing the risk of age-related cognitive decline and dementia, although this remains a topic of debate [6, 7]. Moreover, exercise medicine is effective in alleviating pain and improving physical function through weight loss in individuals with rheumatic and musculoskeletal diseases [8], preventing falls in older adults [9], and treating depression with supervised and group aerobic exercise (AE) of moderate intensity [10]. These results underscore the essential role of exercise medicine in promoting overall human health.

While determining the precise prescription and delivery of exercise to each patient remains challenging due to the lack of accurate information on exercise interventions in previous studies [11], exercise medicine holds promise for enhancing health outcomes, both as a standalone treatment and as a supportive therapy for various diseases, now and in the future.

2. Exercise modalities

Conventional exercise medicine typically involves structured AE and resistance training (RT). However, new exercise modalities have emerged that offer the potential for enhanced effectiveness and efficiency in improving health outcomes.

High-intensity interval training (HIIT) has shown promise as a more effective means of enhancing cardiorespiratory fitness in healthy individuals when compared to traditional AE [12]. It is also similarly effective in improving body composition in overweight and obese adults [13]. Additionally, HIIT exhibits pleiotropic effects, including improvements in cardiorespiratory fitness, physical fitness, muscle strength, cardiac function, mitochondrial citrate synthase activity, and reductions in blood triglycerides and glucose levels in older individuals at risk of sarcopenia [14]. HIIT has proven to be safe, effective, and time-efficient, even in patients with type 2 diabetes [15]. Similarly, sprint interval training, which requires even higher intensity but shorter exercise duration than HIIT, is effective in promoting fat oxidation in overweight or obese individuals [16] and enhances cardiorespiratory fitness and exercise performance in physically active young individuals and athletes [17].

Whole-body vibration has demonstrated benefits, including pain relief and increased knee extensor muscle strength when compared to stretching exercises alone, especially in patients with knee osteoarthritis [18]. It has also shown potential to improve mobility in patients with neurological disorders like stroke and Parkinson's disease [19] and increase bone mineral density in the lumbar spine of postmenopausal women [20].

While the exercise intensity in non-exercise activity thermogenesis (NEAT) and low-intensity resistance exercise with slow movements and tonic force generation (LST) is generally low-to-moderate, and the effects of NEAT and LST may appear relatively modest compared to moderate-to-vigorous intensity exercises, NEAT and LST hold promise in improving health outcomes for patients with chronic diseases [21–28].

Looking ahead, it is likely that new exercise modalities will continue to be developed. Clinicians should remain vigilant and stay informed about these advancements.

3. Technological advancements in exercise medicine

To objectively measure or monitor the PA of individuals, pedometers have been widely used. However, pedometers fall short in accurately measuring the intensity of PA and energy expenditure. To address this issue, accelerometers have emerged as a solution since the 1990s [29]. This technology has steadily advanced, leading to numerous studies exploring the health benefits of light-intensity PA [30]; the relationship between specific PA patterns (such as intensity, bout duration, or frequency) and health outcomes [31]; the relationship between PA, sedentary time (measured by accelerometers), and mortality [32]; and even the detection of concussion episodes

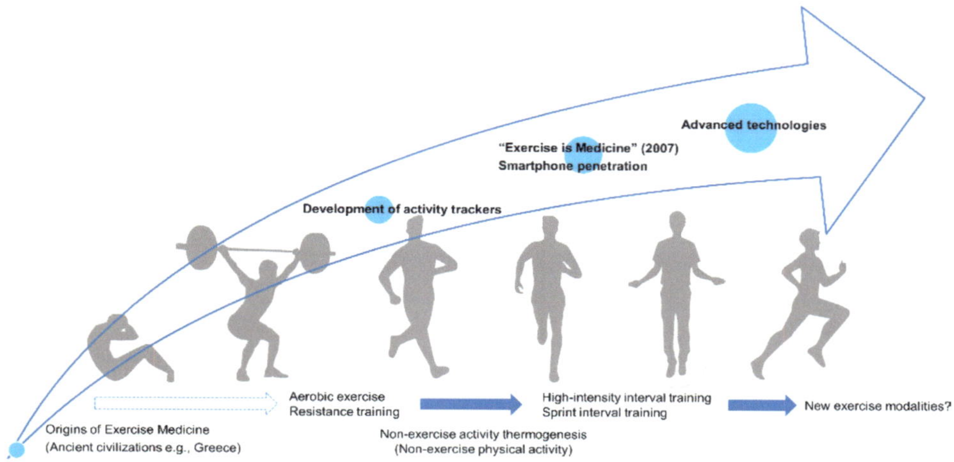

Figure 1.
Past, present, and future of exercise medicine.

in male football players [33]. Today, this technology is regularly incorporated into smartphones [34], enabling people to monitor their daily PA for health management. Furthermore, wearable technologies have proven to be practical and useful in promoting PA in patients with diabetes [35]. The COVID-19 pandemic, which began in 2019, had a detrimental impact on PA and overall health worldwide. If an effective network can be established between healthcare organizations and wearable users, it will also assist people in preventing physical inactivity and health problems during future pandemics [36].

Recently, ChatGPT, a generative artificial intelligence (AI), has significantly impacted the human world and is poised to bring about significant changes in medicine [37]. Within the field of exercise medicine, AI has the potential to effectively promote PA to the same extent as conventional in-person counseling [38]. AI-based interactive exercise has proven more effective in improving cardiorespiratory fitness than conventional gaming exercise, particularly in individuals with obesity [39]. Advanced AI, armed with vast, precise, and practical knowledge about exercise medicine, could provide valuable advice to humans when used appropriately.

Additionally, virtual reality (VR) technology has made remarkable strides. Cardiac rehabilitation using VR enhances exercise capacity, reduces stress and depression, and improves the quality of life [40]. VR exergaming has also shown promise in positively impacting cognitive function in older adults [41]. VR-based exercise therapy can improve upper extremity motor function in patients undergoing rehabilitation after a stroke [42]. VR technologies are expected to play a pivotal role in rehabilitation in the future. Further studies examining the effectiveness of these advanced technologies on health outcomes are warranted.

Figure 1 illustrates the past, present, and future of exercise medicine.

4. New horizons of exercise medicine

This book aims to compile a comprehensive range of effective exercise modalities (from conventional to state-of-the-art) and scientific evidence concerning their impact on health. It also introduces the latest research findings on the biological mechanisms of exercise. Furthermore, it discusses new exercise therapies utilizing cutting-edge scientific technology, explores future possibilities and challenges, and provides recommendations for the advancement of exercise medicine. In my role as an academic editor, I sincerely hope that you, as readers, will enjoy delving into each excellent chapter authored by today's eminent researchers. May you deepen your understanding and find valuable insights for applying exercise medicine in both your daily life and clinical practice.

Acknowledgements

No funding was received to assist with the preparation of this chapter.

Conflict of interest

The author declares no conflict of interest.

Author details

Hidetaka Hamasaki
Hamasaki Clinic, Kagoshima, Japan

*Address all correspondence to: h-hamasaki@umin.ac.jp

References

[1] Toepel T. The doctor in relation to exercise as a factor in medicine and surgery. Atlanta Journal-Record of Medicine. 1907;**9**(2):67-73

[2] Blair SN, Kohl HW 3rd, Paffenbarger RS Jr, Clark DG, Cooper KH, Gibbons LW. Physical fitness and all-cause mortality. A prospective study of healthy men and women. Journal of the American Medical Association. 1989;**262**(17):2395-2401. DOI: 10.1001/jama.262.17.2395

[3] Berryman JW. Exercise is medicine: A historical perspective. Current Sports Medicine Reports. 2010;**9**(4):195-201. DOI: 10.1249/JSR.0b013e3181e7d86d

[4] Fiuza-Luces C, Santos-Lozano A, Joyner M, Carrera-Bastos P, Picazo O, Zugaza JL, et al. Exercise benefits in cardiovasculardisease:Beyondattenuation of traditional risk factors. Nature Reviews. Cardiology. 2018;**15**(12):731-743. DOI: 10.1038/s41569-018-0065-1

[5] Thomas R, Kenfield SA, Yanagisawa Y, Newton RU. Why exercise has a crucial role in cancer prevention, risk reduction and improved outcomes. British Medical Bulletin. 2021;**139**(1):100-119. DOI: 10.1093/bmb/ldab019

[6] Alty J, Farrow M, Lawler K. Exercise and dementia prevention. Practical Neurology. 2020;**20**(3):234-240. DOI: 10.1136/practneurol-2019-002335

[7] Lamb SE, Sheehan B, Atherton N, Nichols V, Collins H, Mistry D, et al. Dementia And Physical Activity (DAPA) trial of moderate to high intensity exercise training for people with dementia: Randomised controlled trial. BMJ. 2018;**361**:k1675. DOI: 10.1136/bmj.k1675

[8] Gwinnutt JM, Wieczorek M, Cavalli G, Balanescu A, Bischoff-Ferrari HA, Boonen A, et al. Effects of physical exercise and body weight on disease-specific outcomes of people with rheumatic and musculoskeletal diseases (RMDs): Systematic reviews and meta-analyses informing the 2021 EULAR recommendations for lifestyle improvements in people with RMDs. RMD Open. 2022;**8**(1):e002168. DOI: 10.1136/rmdopen-2021-002168

[9] Sherrington C, Fairhall N, Kwok W, Wallbank G, Tiedemann A, Michaleff ZA, et al. Evidence on physical activity and falls prevention for people aged 65+ years: Systematic review to inform the WHO guidelines on physical activity and sedentary behaviour. International Journal of Behavioral Nutrition and Physical Activity. 2020;**17**(1):144. DOI: 10.1186/s12966-020-01041-3

[10] Heissel A, Heinen D, Brokmeier LL, Skarabis N, Kangas M, Vancampfort D, et al. Exercise as medicine for depressive symptoms? A systematic review and meta-analysis with meta-regression. British Journal of Sports Medicine. 2023;**57**(16):1049-1057. DOI: 10.1136/bjsports-2022-106282

[11] Hansford HJ, Wewege MA, Cashin AG, Hagstrom AD, Clifford BK, McAuley JH, et al. If exercise is medicine, why don't we know the dose? An overview of systematic reviews assessing reporting quality of exercise interventions in health and disease. British Journal of Sports Medicine. 2022;**56**(12):692-700. DOI: 10.1136/bjsports-2021-104977

[12] Milanović Z, Sporiš G, Weston M. Effectiveness of high-intensity interval

training (HIT) and continuous endurance training for VO2max improvements: A systematic review and meta-analysis of controlled trials. Sports Medicine. 2015;**45**(10):1469-1481. DOI: 10.1007/s40279-015-0365-0

[13] Wewege M, van den Berg R, Ward RE, Keech A. The effects of high-intensity interval training vs. moderate-intensity continuous training on body composition in overweight and obese adults: A systematic review and meta-analysis. Obesity Reviews. 2017;**18**(6):635-646. DOI: 10.1111/obr.12532

[14] Wu ZJ, Wang ZY, Gao HE, Zhou XF, Li FH. Impact of high-intensity interval training on cardiorespiratory fitness, body composition, physical fitness, and metabolic parameters in older adults: A meta-analysis of randomized controlled trials. Experimental Gerontology. 2021;**150**:111345. DOI: 10.1016/j.exger.2021.111345

[15] Hamasaki H. Interval exercise therapy for type 2 diabetes. Current Diabetes Reviews. 2018;**14**(2):129-137. DOI: 10.2174/1573399812666161101103655

[16] Atakan MM, Guzel Y, Shrestha N, Kosar SN, Grgic J, Astorino TA, et al. Effects of high-intensity interval training (HIIT) and sprint interval training (SIT) on fat oxidation during exercise: A systematic review and meta-analysis. British Journal of Sports Medicine. 2022;**56**. DOI: 10.1136/bjsports-2021-105181

[17] Boullosa D, Dragutinovic B, Feuerbacher JF, Benítez-Flores S, Coyle EF, Schumann M. Effects of short sprint interval training on aerobic and anaerobic indices: A systematic review and meta-analysis. Scandinavian Journal of Medicine & Science in Sports. 2022;**32**(5):810-820. DOI: 10.1111/sms.14133

[18] Qiu CG, Chui CS, Chow SKH, Cheung WH, Wong RMY. Effects of whole-body vibration therapy on knee osteoarthritis: A systematic review and meta-analysis of randomized controlled trials. Journal of Rehabilitation Medicine. 2022;**54**:jrm00266. DOI: 10.2340/jrm.v54.2032

[19] Alashram AR, Padua E, Annino G. Effects of whole-body vibration on motor impairments in patients with neurological disorders: A systematic review. American Journal of Physical Medicine & Rehabilitation. 2019;**98**(12):1084-1098. DOI: 10.1097/PHM.0000000000001252

[20] Marín-Cascales E, Alcaraz PE, Ramos-Campo DJ, Martinez-Rodriguez A, Chung LH, Rubio-Arias JÁ. Whole-body vibration training and bone health in postmenopausal women: A systematic review and meta-analysis. Medicine (Baltimore). 2018;**97**(34):e11918. DOI: 10.1097/MD.0000000000011918

[21] Hamasaki H, Yanai H, Mishima S, Mineyama T, Yamamoto-Honda R, Kakei M, et al. Correlations of non-exercise activity thermogenesis to metabolic parameters in Japanese patients with type 2 diabetes. Diabetology and Metabolic Syndrome. 2013;**5**(1):26. DOI: 10.1186/1758-5996-5-26

[22] Hamasaki H, Yanai H, Kakei M, Ezaki O, Noda M. Non-exercise activity thermogenesis is associated with markers for diabetic microangiopathy in Japanese female patients with type 2 diabetes. International Journal of Cardiology. 2013;**168**(5):4836-4837. DOI: 10.1016/j.ijcard.2013.07.004

[23] Hamasaki H, Yanai H, Kakei M, Noda M, Ezaki O. Higher daily energy expenditure by locomotive activities is favorably associated with cardiac

autonomic nervous function and arterial stiffness. International Journal of Cardiology. 2015;**194**:70-71. DOI: 10.1016/j.ijcard.2015.05.094

[24] Hamasaki H, Noda M, Moriyama S, Yoshikawa R, Katsuyama H, Sako A, et al. Daily physical activity assessed by a Triaxial accelerometer is beneficially associated with waist circumference, serum triglycerides, and insulin resistance in Japanese patients with prediabetes or untreated early type 2 diabetes. Journal Diabetes Research. 2015;**2015**:526201. DOI: 10.1155/2015/526201

[25] Hamasaki H, Kawashima Y, Tamada Y, Furuta M, Katsuyama H, Sako A, et al. Associations of low-intensity resistance training with body composition and lipid profile in obese patients with type 2 diabetes. PLoS One. 2015;**10**(7):e0132959. DOI: 10.1371/journal.pone.0132959

[26] Hamasaki H, Yanai H, Kakei M, Noda M, Ezaki O. The association between daily physical activity and plasma B-type natriuretic peptide in patients with glucose intolerance: A cross-sectional study. BMJ Open. 2015;**5**(1):e006276. DOI: 10.1136/bmjopen-2014-006276

[27] Hamasaki H, Ezaki O, Yanai H. Nonexercise activity thermogenesis is significantly lower in type 2 diabetic patients with mental disorders than in those without mental disorders: A cross-sectional study. Medicine (Baltimore). 2016;**95**(2):e2517. DOI: 10.1097/MD.0000000000002517

[28] Shoji T, Hamasaki H, Kawaguchi A, Waragai Y, Yanai H. Effects of low-intensity resistance exercise with slow movement and tonic force generation on short-term glycemic variability in healthy subjects: A randomized controlled study. Applied Sciences. 2021;**11**(4):1536. DOI: 10.3390/app11041536

[29] Bassett DR, Troiano RP, McClain JJ, Wolff DL. Accelerometer-based physical activity: Total volume per day and standardized measures. Medicine and Science in Sports and Exercise. 2015;**47**(4):833-838. DOI: 10.1249/MSS.0000000000000468

[30] Füzéki E, Engeroff T, Banzer W. Health benefits of light-intensity physical activity: A systematic review of accelerometer data of the National Health and Nutrition Examination Survey (NHANES). Sports Medicine. 2017;**47**(9):1769-1793. DOI: 10.1007/s40279-017-0724-0

[31] Brady R, Brown WJ, Hillsdon M, Mielke GI. Patterns of accelerometer-measured physical activity and health outcomes in adults: A systematic review. Medicine and Science in Sports and Exercise. 2022;**54**(7):1155-1166. DOI: 10.1249/MSS.0000000000002900

[32] Ekelund U, Tarp J, Steene-Johannessen J, Hansen BH, Jefferis B, Fagerland MW, et al. Dose-response associations between accelerometry measured physical activity and sedentary time and all cause mortality: Systematic review and harmonised meta-analysis. BMJ. 2019;**366**:l4570. DOI: 10.1136/bmj.l4570

[33] Brennan JH, Mitra B, Synnot A, McKenzie J, Willmott C, McIntosh AS, et al. Accelerometers for the assessment of concussion in male athletes: A systematic review and meta-analysis. Sports Medicine. 2017;**47**(3):469-478. DOI: 10.1007/s40279-016-0582-1

[34] Higgins JP. Smartphone applications for patients' health and fitness. The American Journal of Medicine. 2016;**129**(1):11-19. DOI: 10.1016/j.amjmed.2015.05.038

[35] Hamasaki H. Efficacy of wearable devices to measure and promote physical activity in the management of diabetes. EMJ Diabetes. 2018;**6**(1):62-69. DOI: 10.33590/emjdiabet/10312817

[36] Hamasaki H. Daily physical activity and sleep measured by wearable activity trackers during the coronavirus disease 2019 pandemic: A lesson for preventing physical inactivity during future pandemics. Applied Sciences. 2021;**11**(21):9956. DOI: 10.3390/app11219956

[37] Eysenbach G. The role of ChatGPT, generative language models, and artificial intelligence in medical education: A conversation with ChatGPT and a call for papers. JMIR Medical Education. 2023;**9**:e46885. DOI: 10.2196/46885

[38] Oh YJ, Zhang J, Fang ML, Fukuoka Y. A systematic review of artificial intelligence chatbots for promoting physical activity, healthy diet, and weight loss. International Journal of Behavioral Nutrition and Physical Activity. 2021;**18**(1):160. DOI: 10.1186/s12966-021-01224-6

[39] Oh W, An Y, Min S, Park C. Comparative effectiveness of artificial intelligence-based interactive home exercise applications in adolescents with obesity. Sensors (Basel). 2022;**22**(19):7352. DOI: 10.3390/s22197352

[40] Chen Y, Cao L, Xu Y, Zhu M, Guan B, Ming WK. Effectiveness of virtual reality in cardiac rehabilitation: A systematic review and meta-analysis of randomized controlled trials. International Journal of Nursing Studies. 2022;**133**:104323. DOI: 10.1016/j.ijnurstu.2022.104323

[41] Yen HY, Chiu HL. Virtual reality exergames for improving older Adults' cognition and depression: A systematic review and meta-analysis of randomized control trials. Journal of the American Medical Directors Association. 2021;**22**(5):995-1002. DOI: 10.1016/j.jamda.2021.03.009

[42] Chen J, Or CK, Chen T. Effectiveness of using virtual reality-supported exercise therapy for upper extremity motor rehabilitation in patients with stroke: Systematic review and meta-analysis of randomized controlled trials. Journal of Medical Internet Research. 2022;**24**(6):e24111. DOI: 10.2196/24111

Chapter 2

Exercise Is Medicine through Time: Prescription of Adapted Physical Activity in Treatment and Rehabilitation

Katerina Asonitou, Soteria Yiannaki and Dimitra Koutsouki

Abstract

The history of physical activity and sport dates to ancient times, when it was not only a means of preparation for military readiness but also had religious and educational purposes. The relationship between physical activity and good health goes back centuries accepted, as formulated by Hippocrates 2500 years ago. In Greek antiquity, "*gymnastike*" highlighted physical beauty in harmony with the soul and spirit, perfecting simultaneously an individual's personality and health. Lifelong exercise administered by gymnasts was applied to strengthen weak limbs, and contributed to the healing of patients when applied in the healthcare facilities of the time, as mentioned in "Asclepieia." Nowadays, the idea that "exercise is medicine" has two components: (1) every patient's treatment or rehabilitation plan should include physical activity and exercise training, but the prescription must be tailored to the patient's specific needs and (2) doctors' challenge lies in implementing this medical prescription for adapted physical activity (APA), which encourages patients to lead more active lives.

Keywords: physical activity history, adapted exercise training, prescription, treatment, adaptive exercise, chronic disease, rehabilitation, lifestyle habits

1. Introduction

According to Barbin [1], the term "adapted PA" (physical and sports activities) refers to any physical activity or sport that is modified and tailored to a person's functional movement, restrictions, contraindications to certain exercises, and surroundings in order to provide a means of participation for those with a variety of disabilities or long-term medical conditions. Additionally, APA is frequently employed by medical practitioners as a rehabilitation strategy for social and educational engagement, reeducation, community reintegration, and the avoidance of secondary disorders [1].

Thornton et al. [2] have proposed that a cost-effective strategy for promoting physical activity (PA) would be to prescribe PA as part of primary healthcare. To

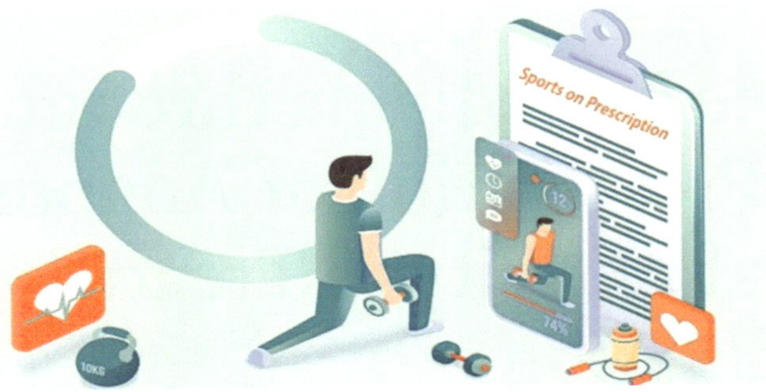

Figure 1.
Impact of "sports on prescription" on the health and well-being of patients [4].

guarantee appropriate PA prescription, individuals with disabilities must have their unique requirements, capacities, and indications considered when prescribing PA. Nonetheless, to guarantee appropriate PA prescription, the demands, capacities, and symptoms of everyone with a disability must be taken into account. Sedentary behavior among people with disabilities has been found to be influenced by both personal and environmental factors, such as pain, lack of energy, and self-consciousness about exercising in public. Personal factors include things such as pain, lack of exercise equipment, social exclusion, and inadequately trained and resourced health staff. For people of all ages, research clearly shows the advantages of maintaining an active lifestyle across a variety of physical and mental health concerns. The Department of Health and Human Services in the United States offers precise recommendations for physical exercise at various phases of life. Some recommendations and things to think about are included on this website [3] for persons who are pregnant, elderly, or have chronic health issues. Also, it is important to inform our doctor about the sort of activity we want to begin whether we are a new fitness enthusiast or have a particular medical issue. For a particular health issue, they might check the format to make sure it is safe (**Figure 1**).

2. Exercise and 'well-being': from the past to the present

2.1 Exercise, health, and illness in antiquity

Movement constitutes the characteristic feature of life [5] and is considered an innate disposition of humans. Exercise consists of movements that, when applied, benefit both the body and the soul [5]. Games, physical activity, physical culture activities, and competitions found expression in the cultures of antiquity following the customs and culture they developed.

In those cultures, exercise was seen as essential for maintaining a healthy state and preventing diseases. Ancient Chinese culture placed importance on health and well-being through various practices. Practices such as qigong (breathing exercises) and yoga were used as forms of exercise to promote physical and mental health. In ancient India, while physical exercise was recognized and practiced, the focus was more on general physical activities rather than a structured exercise prescription for health purposes. In Greek antiquity, a strong emphasis was placed on physical fitness and exercise for maintaining a healthy body and mind [6].

In the ancient Greek world, the art of healing and preserving life was subject to the laws of the universe and protected by the Gods. Health, the daughter of the god Asclepius [7], is deified as people realized the importance of preserving and treating diseases, and Asclepieia existed scattered throughout the Hellenic territory. In classical antiquity, health was considered a harmonious state of body and soul. The central concept was the idea of balance and harmony of the individual, aiming for well-being, resulting in the development of a holistic approach to health and disease through exercise. Some representative beliefs of physicians and philosophers are cited below.

Hippocrates (460–377 BC) transformed hieratic or theocratic medicine into a rational discipline. In the works of the Hippocratic Corpus, it is argued that health depends on the balance between diet and exercise. Hippocratic physicians believed that physical well-being can only be achieved through appropriate education, with moderation adapted to the individual's condition, age, and strength, which should avoid excess. They were opposed to both excessive athletic training and the avoidance of exercise, as well as to gluttony [8].

The fundamental layout of the Asclepieion in Kos indicates Hippocrates' belief in a comprehensive healthcare model. In his school, scientific principles were combined with pharmaceutical treatment, dietary plans, and both physical and mental exercises, along with divine intervention. Additionally, at the Asclepieion of Kos, every patient received a comprehensive treatment regimen that incorporated physical activities, massages, and walks deemed essential for the restoration of health, the well-being of the soul, and inner peace [9].

Both physical and psychospiritual education became central interests, and Plato (427–347 BC), influenced by Socrates and Hippocrates, defined that proper education is divided into the education of the body and the education of the soul, the former being called gymnastics and the latter music. Consequently, the lessons corresponding to gymnastics and music were divided into physical perfection and mental well-being. Physical education was closely linked to psychospiritual education, so citizens should engage in physical exercise for life. According to Plato, good physical condition is shaped by gymnastics, the art that preserves health and physical disposition through proper diet and rules, and medicine, which operates therapeutically. The purpose of gymnastics is the improvement of bodies through physical care, as determined by the right reason. In his work "Timaeus," he describes the result of the harmonious movement of body and soul: "From both these evils the one means of salvation is this—neither to exercise the soul without the body nor the body without the soul, so that they may be evenly matched and sound of health. Thus the student of mathematics, or of any other subject, who works very hard with his intellect must also provide his body with exercise by practicing gymnastics; while he who is diligent in molding his body must, in turn, provide his soul with motion by cultivating music and philosophy in general, if either is to deserve to be called truly both beautiful and virtuous: kalos kagathos" [10].

The attainment of eudaimonia was synonymous with balance, so health and illness, virtue and vice, were consequences of the symmetry or asymmetry of the soul to the body. Thus, the soul should not move without the body, nor the body without the soul, and both should be cared for to maintain balance and health. People should be educated in gymnastics from childhood and throughout their lives [11].

According to Aristotle (384–323 BC), "to act well and to live well" was the primary pursuit, meaning human happiness (eudaimonia). This happiness could be achieved through the harmony of the body. He considered gymnastics as the science of "moderation in pains" and thus distinguished athletic exertion from physical activity that contributed to the individual's balance, provided it did not involve excessive or inappropriate exercises. Thus, the art of health was preserved [12].

Philological evidence from the Roman Imperial period indicates that intellectuals of that era redefined gymnastics in connection to medicine and the pursuit of well-being, aligning with the classic beliefs of Greek antiquity [13].

In the texts of Plutarch (46–120 AD), his belief in gymnastics is recorded, which, through appropriate exercises, ensures health and cultivates military readiness. The purpose of gymnastics was the well-being of the body, while medicine aimed at maintaining health. Exercises should not be exhaustive or specialized. The usefulness of gymnastics relates to the harmony and strength of the body, while when taken to excess or pursued for competitive goals, it becomes an obstacle to the spiritual development of young people [14].

The physician Galen (128–200 AD) defined that not every movement is exercise, only active movement, and set the criterion as the alteration of the normal rhythm of breathing. He urged those who exercised for health reasons not to overstrain themselves to avoid the psychosomatic dependence caused by athletes' exercise. He recognized the connection between well-being and gymnastics and the preservation of health through gymnastics, as well as the therapeutic dimension of both medicine and gymnastics [15].

According to Philostratus (179–249 AD), gymnastics was created from the synthesis of the art of paidotribai and medicine but was more comprehensive than the former and a part of the latter. Suitable exercise could remove excess flesh and fat from the body, soften a hardened limb, or strengthen or warm the body. Gymnastics, along with appropriate diet and rubbing, could stop colds, excessive sweating, and wasting, which doctors treated with therapeutic measures [16].

Ancient Greek culture perceived health as a balanced state between exercise and diet. Hippocratic physicians promoted physical well-being through proper education and moderation in exercise, contrary to excess or avoidance. Plato and other philosophers considered gymnastics an integral part of education, promoting balance between body and soul. Similarly, well-being was regarded as a result of the harmony between body and spirit. With gymnastics being a "guardian" of health, exercise preserved and cultivated health while also preventing and treating illness.

2.2 From practice to theory and from theory to knowledge

The "gymnast" – the educated physical trainer – represented the evolution of the paidotribe (who dealt with gymnastics issues utilizing his experience and practical knowledge as a former athlete). Until the distinction of their competencies, there was a period when the two terms were used interchangeably.

Plato, in his work "Republic" refers to the paidotribe-gymnast Herodicus, who: "... was a paidotribe and became a valetudinarian, and blended gymnastics and medicine, for the torment first and chiefly of himself and then of many successors," introducing therapeutic gymnastics. The knowledge of the paidotribe-gymnast is comparable to that of a physician, and one should equally take their comments seriously. Both are specialists for the body and can discern a patient. The two arts, gymnastics and medicine, thus the gymnasts and the physicians, can properly distinguish (possess the appropriate knowledge) the types of purification performed on living organisms. They also knew about diets and applied suitable nutrition. Therefore, we can understand that there was a period when the boundaries between the two were indistinct [17].

Over time, the gymnast acquired knowledge such as anatomy, physiology, pedagogy, the art of physiognomy (psychology), knew different exercises, and simultaneously the result of the exercises on the trainee; he can be characterized as a 'pentathlete of knowledge' [18]. At the peak of his scientific status, he could apply the appropriate exercises for training, rehabilitation, restoration, cultivation, and preservation of health.

2.3 The modern past: exercise is medicine

In the introduction of his paper, Berryman [19] highlights the pivotal significance of the texts of Hippocrates and Galen, referring to the stimulus that influenced the formation of the physical education movement in the nineteenth century. Specifically, he notes the context of the "six things nonnatural" (air, diet sleep and wake, exercise and rest, excretions and retentions, and passion of the mind). If the nonnaturals were observed and practiced in moderation, health would be the result.

Exercise was incorporated into the regimen, hygiene, and preventive medicine literature in the late nineteenth century and was primarily used for prophylaxis. It was recommended as a treatment for various ailments and was considered part of medicine. In New York, 1806, physician Shadrach Ricketson published "Means of Preserving Health and Preventing Diseases," which discussed the negative effects of idleness and luxury on health and the importance of exercise.

In 1880, physicians took on leadership roles in physical education associations and published corresponding journals, oversaw gyms, gave lectures, and prescribed exercise. In 1900, the course of medicine began to change, emphasizing research, vaccines, and the scientific specialization of physicians. Later on, the Harvard Fatigue Laboratory (1930s–40s) conducted groundbreaking studies on exercise, laying the foundation for exercise science research in the 1960s.

Meanwhile, there was a shift in physical education from a focus on health and exercise led by physicians to a games and sports curriculum led by coaches. The new sports doctrine emphasized citizenship, teamwork, character, democratic living, and sportsmanship, but it was found that the health of millions of Americans had problems. It was reaffirmed that physical activity was a fundamental characteristic of health. In the 1970s, exercise entered people's lives as a lifestyle, and in the following years, magazines and books were published connecting exercise with health. In 2007, the American Medical Association and American College of Sports Medicine inaugurated the Exercise is Medicine health initiative, making the culture of exercise and health in Greek antiquity come to life once more.

3. Medical usage of adapted physical activity (APA)

3.1 Exercise as medication for treating many chronic diseases

A five-year Swedish primary care study conducted by Joelsson and colleagues [20] investigates the effects of long-term prescription physical exercise on individuals who are physically inactive and have metabolic risk factors. The intervention involved prescriptions for tailored physical exercise together with follow-ups, which increased engagement and motivation. In fifteen basic healthcare clinics in Gothenburg, Sweden, individual interviews were subjected to a qualitative content analysis after a purposeful selection of interview participants. Ten patients responded to the intervention, whereas the remaining ten patients did not, for a total of twenty physically inactive individuals with one or more metabolic syndrome components. The patients' mean age ranged from 25 to 73 years.

Three different impact groups were identified by the interviews. First, personal modifications led to a rise in physical activity. Second, maintaining and setting priorities for lifestyle modifications was made easier with the help of follow-up and support. Third, patients may be more motivated if they have control over their treatment and see results. Personalized physical exercise on prescription with frequent follow-ups can help to enhance and sustain motivation and physical activity levels.

In conclusion, physical activity levels were observed to rise with individually prescribed physical exercise for inactive adults with the metabolic syndrome. Patients exhibited more motivation when they created their own physical activity plans. Healthcare professionals' support and follow-up made lifestyle changes priority, and experiences with positive health outcomes contributed to maintaining or increasing levels of physical activity.

Pedersen & Saltin [21] conducted a systematic review study that looked at the most recent evidence-based basis for prescribing exercise as medicine in the treatment of 26 different diseases: cancer; metabolic diseases (obesity, hyperlipidemia, metabolic syndrome, polycystic ovarian syndrome, type 2 diabetes, and type 1 diabetes); pulmonary diseases (chronic obstructive pulmonary disease, asthma, and cystic fibrosis); musculoskeletal disorders (osteoarthritis, osteoporosis, back pain, and rheumatoid arthritis); and psychological diseases (dementia, Parkinson's disease, multiple sclerosis, dementia, polycystic ovarian syndrome, type 2 diabetes, type 1 diabetes, and cerebral apoplexy). Exercise therapy's impact on the etiology and symptoms of disease is described, along with potential mechanisms of action. They have provided the reader with the finest advice for the type and amount of exercise that should be advised for each condition after analyzing the scientific literature.

According to the authors' conclusion, it is customary in the medical field to recommend the evidence-based course of therapy that is most likely to be successful and have the fewest risks or adverse effects. According to the available data, exercise therapy may be more beneficial than medical treatment in some circumstances or may even enhance its effects in others. Now that so much knowledge has been gathered, it must be put into practice. It's time for the health systems to put in place the necessary framework to guarantee that supervised exercise can be prescribed as medicine, even though there is still work to be done in defining the best kind and amount of exercise and investigating whether one-legged training, high-intensity interval training, or other more recent exercise modalities which will be appropriate for certain diagnoses.

Furthermore, it is critical that society encourages an active lifestyle. When you advise people to move, they do not. When the situation demands it, they shift. Accessibility is crucial to raising a population's level of physical activity. Laws and political declarations on "health consequences" are necessary. Politicians should always consider concerns related to gender and ethnicity, but they should also take into account health-related issues, such as how design and infrastructure may affect how physically active a community is.

The goal of a cross-sectional study [22] conducted between February 2020 and July 2021 at the Nancy University Center of Sports Medicine and APA, France, was to determine the heart rate and level of exercise intensity in a sample of 71 patients with chronic illnesses who were not using beta-blockers from the departments of hematology, rheumatology, obesity, and other specialties who were taking part in a hospital-based adaptive physical activity program (APA). Physiotherapists and exercise specialists with academic degrees in adapted physical activity (APA) typically collaborate to offer APA in hospital settings. The APA program was customized for each patient, taking into account their expectations, psychological characteristics, physical fitness, and preferred forms of exercise.

A mean age of 42.6 and a mean BMI of 36.7 (±10.6) were found in the 52 female patients. About 57.3% of the patients had been referred because of obesity. There were 36 individuals with impaired exercise performance and 39 patients with normal exercise capacity. Prior to engaging in a supervised APA practice, the participants methodically completed a cardiopulmonary exercise test; heart rate (HR) was monitored during the first session via a telemetry wireless device. Drawing from the outcomes of the functional assessment of exercise performance examined two patient groups: (1) unrestricted exercise performance (maximal oxygen uptake exceeding 80% of the theoretical reference) and (2) restricted exercise performance (maximum oxygen uptake falling short of 80% of the theoretical value).

Patients in both groups had HRs that were higher than 70% of their true maximal HR during the most intense 15-minute APA session episode. Researchers found that people with a range of chronic illnesses had modest levels of APA exercise intensity. In terms of exercise intensity, they did not see any significant differences in the patients' capacities—that is, between those with and without a maximum performance restriction. 69.2% of maximum capacity was the mean and median actual intensity level of exercise during hospital-based APA sessions among a sample of patients. The highest level of intensity (75.8% of maximum capacity) was only achieved during the most intense 15 minutes. The findings emphasize the need for a preventative functional evaluation of cardiopulmonary fitness in patients with fragile chronic conditions prior to prescribing any exercise, as intense activity is known to increase cardiovascular events.

However, it is critical to acknowledge the significance of exercise professionals in order to integrate them into the global healthcare strategy and secure their support. The findings consequently emphasize the critical role that medical practitioners play in both systematically assessing patients' health state and encouraging frequent physical exercise in them. To facilitate a shift toward a less sedentary and more independent lifestyle, healthcare practitioners often prioritize patient-centered dialog, individualized physical activity recommendations accompanied by written prescriptions, and follow-up throughout patient treatment. The findings indicate that medical practitioners ought to carefully assess each patient's condition of health, given the increased stress levels that accompany exercise. This will increase the efficacy of the WHO slogan for 2018–2030, *"More active people for a healthier world."*

There are restrictions on this study. Firstly, any expansion of the results is impossible due to the sample size; a single medical center's small sample of 75 APA practitioners participated in the study. Furthermore, a subgroup analysis of several chronic diseases was hampered by the high proportion of obese people. Consequently, HR has limits even if it is the most practical metric for assessing the intensity in an ecological setting. However, the HR curve is influenced by age, gender, and performance, among other factors.

This study investigated high levels of exercise intensity (>70% of HRpeak in exercise tests) in individuals with and without performance limitations who were suffering from various chronic conditions. The study's primary strength is its novelty, as it allowed us to capture the real practice intensity throughout APA sessions using physiological data that were collected. In this study, individual capabilities and progressive exercise tests are included. In fact, VO2max is the gold standard for evaluating a patient's functional abilities. Nonetheless, long-term research analyzing a broader sample would clarify these findings. The results show that safe exercise routines may be developed, and medical risk can be assessed by creating personalized exercise plans that are appropriate for the patient's present health status [22].

4. Adaptive exercise prescription for special populations

4.1 People with brain impairment

An important loss or anomaly in the anatomy of the brain is called brain impairment (BI). Brain damage can result from a variety of medical diseases, such as stroke, traumatic brain injury, and cerebral palsy. Studies reveal that individuals with brain injury (BI) participate in much less physical activity compared to those without BI. The loss of muscular strength, flexibility, and cardiovascular fitness resulting from physical inactivity may worsen the secondary impairment. Furthermore, because BI patients tend to be highly sedentary, it has been proposed that they are more vulnerable to conditions including cancer, hypertension, myocardial infarction, chronic obstructive pulmonary disease, anxiety, and depression—all conditions associated with physical inactivity. Crucially, research indicates that increased physical activity can help people with BI improve a variety of indices, including as muscular strength, functional independence, and cardiorespiratory fitness [23]. Therefore, it is critical to plan and evaluate interventions that successfully promote physical activity participation in people with brain injuries.

A health professional with expertise in organized exercise prescription for people with disabilities, encouraging community involvement for people with disabilities, and utilizing evidence-based techniques for physical activity promotion is delivering the program. People go through Steps 1, 2, 3, and 4 in around ten in-person meetings spread out over a 12-week period. Each session lasts around 1 hour, and the intervals between sessions are customized based on the needs of the individual. As community access is arranged, skills are learned, habits are developed, and discussions on values, motivation, and physical activity involvement evolve; more sessions are often completed in the first 6 weeks [23].

Apart from the face-to-face sessions, Steps 2 and 3 also involve electronic notifications, emails, or reminder calls to reaffirm the session's objectives and/or act as a catalyst for additional action (e.g., to talk about a participant's first community exercise class or a prompt to contact a nearby sports club). How much use is made of these tactics will depend on the participant's impairment profile (especially memory impairment), preferences, availability, and capacity for employing various communication strategies.

A community-based rehabilitation paradigm is used to provide the APAP. Services offered in a person's home or community—that is, the actual surroundings they usually reside in or have easy access to—are referred to as community-based rehabilitation. To facilitate program replication and improvement for clinical practice, this document provides a thorough explanation of the program's components together with a real case study example for researchers and practitioners to review. The purpose of presenting these elements is to help researchers and practitioners understand what information/knowledge and abilities are required in order to integrate the program into clinical practice [23].

This article outlines a community-based, specially designed program to encourage persons with BI to participate in physical exercise. It has been demonstrated that the program works well to encourage individuals with BI to undertake physical exercise. In contrast to previously assessed programs, the APAP stands out for its extensive pre-participation assessment that is mapped against the ICF domains to customize the program to everyone's health, personal preferences, and environmental factors; it also uses a community-based rehabilitation model rather than providing care in a fixed facility and the application of specialized behavior modification techniques in addition to regimented exercise prescription and lifestyle physical activity engagement. Because customized community-based physical activity programs are associated with sustained physical activity participation, and they are inexpensive to administer, they are a good choice.

4.2 People with intellectual disabilities (ID)

Pre- and post-exercise intervention programs were evaluated by Asonitou and colleagues [24], who also looked at two other components of adult ID. The intervention and control groups differed from one another, and the two groups can become significantly different after the intervention program depending on two factors. The intervention group was expected to show improved anthropometry features and higher levels of physical fitness after a four-month training session.

The study comprised 38 adults with intellectual impairments who were split into two groups: the intervention group (n = 19) which underwent exercise training and the control group (n = 19) which did not get any exercise training. While the control group had no instruction and was just instructed to maintain their regular physical activity, the intervention group underwent an intense 16-week exercise program. Over the course of four consecutive months (16-week), the exercise intervention program was carried out twice a week. Every week, there were two 60-minute training sessions that included a range of motor tasks aimed at improving endurance, balance, coordination, speed, and muscular strength.

The testing was placed in the gym or courtyard of the daily care and training center, which met all facility requirements (health and sanitary standards, enough space, lighting, right flooring, enough equipment, accessories, and measuring tools). Although a few individuals required help to complete the tasks, none of the participants left the sessions early. The adapted physical education teachers led each training session, and the investigator supervised any interventions [24].

In order to encourage a more active and healthy way of life, the study demonstrated that adults with mild intellectual disabilities can benefit from a structural physical exercise program in terms of their physical fitness, particularly in terms of muscle strength and endurance, balance, flexibility, speed, and cardio-respiratory endurance as well as anthropometry characteristics such as weight, fat, and BMI.

This shows that persons with moderate ID can benefit from structured physical activity and a tailored training program as an effective intervention to increase their level of fitness. Therefore, more physical activity would enable people with ID to engage in community outdoor activities, foster integration with people without disabilities, and increase their physical fitness, so they can handle daily tasks more easily and lead healthier and more fulfilling lives.

4.3 Child obesity

The evidence-based intervention known as physical activity on prescription (PAP) has been found to have positive effects on adult physical activity levels in Swedish primary healthcare centers. It is crucial to address physical inactivity from an early age as it is a major contributing factor to childhood obesity, which is correlated with adult obesity. Bernhardsson and her colleagues [25] investigated the implementation of the PAP on obese children. This project's main twofold goal was to assess (a) children's, parents', and healthcare professionals' experiences with PAP and (b) the requirements, necessary conditions, factors, and viability of using PAP tailored to children with obesity in pediatric healthcare.

Swedish primary healthcare practitioners have identified two obstacles to adopting PAP for adults: a lack of organizational support and a lack of understanding about the intervention. Positive attitudes among coworkers and both local and central support networks are facilitators. It is important to include parents in any efforts to encourage physical activity as family support and parental role models are critical for children when adopting physical exercise [25].

Managers and medical staff from 26 pediatric clinics in Region Västra Götaland, Sweden, were invited to participate in an online survey during the study's initial phase. A portion of this sample was used in a focus group investigation. PAP was customized to the target audience and circumstance based on the inferences made from these two pieces of data. In the second phase of the clinical research, 60 obese (ISO-BMI > 30) children between the ages of six and twelve, together with one of their parents or legal guardians, took part. The purpose of the study was to assess the personalized PAP intervention. The implementation process and clinical outcomes were assessed both before and after the intervention, as well as at the 8 and 12-month follow-ups. The four fundamental ideas of the Normalization Process Theory are implementation results; coherence, cognitive engagement, group work, and reflexive monitoring; as well as the suitability, practicality, and acceptability of the PAP intervention. Adherence, dosage, intervention fidelity, recruitment and retention rates, and other process outcomes are included. Clinical outcomes include BMI, metabolic risk factors, sleep, health-related quality of life, self-efficacy, and desire for physical activity in addition to patterns of physical activity. Finally, we will use semi-structured interviews to examine the viewpoints of kids and parents. The Normalization Process Theory served as the foundation for the investigations' design and analysis [25].

Through this study, new information will be available on whether PAP is feasible for obese children as well as if and how evidence-based interventions may be implemented and modified for use with different populations and circumstances.

4.4 Breast cancer survivors (multidisciplinary approach)

The international literature emphasizes the importance of physical activity (PA) in the first steps after cancer surgery. The regular practice of physical exercise causes positive adaptations in several functional capacities, with positive consequences on patients' quality of life. This study was designed to assess the impact of a post-operative training program on the functional abilities and quality of life of breast cancer (BC) survivors. The protocol was tailored to account for both cancer-related difficulties and the existence of comorbidities [26].

The collaboration of sport medicine doctors (who prescribe exercise and do risk assessment), kinesiologists (who train), and oncologists (who recommend patients) proved essential. A group of 35 post-surgery BC patients voluntarily chose to participate in either the Usual Care Group (UC Group) or an online Adapted PA (APA) program twice a week for 4 months. The results showed that the APA Group's functional capacity rose by 13.1% ($p = 0.000$), while their perceived effort reduced by 19.7% ($p = 0.020$). Within the same cohort, there was a significant increase ($p = 0.050$) in the overall health as assessed by the EORTC-QLQ-C30 questionnaire. In the UC Group, no differences were discovered. Operation Phalco, which established a network of kinesiologists, sports medicine specialists, and oncologists, reaffirms the need to plan a post-operative course in which APA ought to be included in cancer patient care from the outset [26].

Based on the positive physiological and psychological outcomes that Schutz et al. have shown in BC survivors, the method could be able to overcome the PA barriers related to lack of individualization [27, 28]. To be more specific, the study's results showed that the patient's overall health status had improved because the patient felt less tired during the test and had a higher functional capacity as determined by the 6MWT, a test that assesses general health in BC patients. Skeletal muscular deconditioning is one among the main adverse consequences of BC [29].

Increased muscular strength may be a general predictor of functional lower limb strength and improved balance. The APA group demonstrated this by increasing the load lifted in the 1RM leg press and the number of repetitions completed during the 30" STS test [30, 31]. Otherwise, there were no appreciable changes in APA as indicated by the upper limb strength testing. This might occur because of the restricted overloads employed during the 4-month intervention (1–3 kg) and the fact that the exercise routine was delivered via video conference, which required the exercises to be safe. Furthermore, rather than focusing on increasing strength, "PHALCO" training was designed to restore the function of the operated limb. The findings showed that, even in a pandemic scenario, a multidisciplinary and integrated strategy including oncologists, sport doctors, and APA kinesiologists is safe and practicable during the post-operative BC period and can enhance the quality of life for these patients. Additionally, there were no unfavorable incidents or dropout rates during training sessions for the APA group.

"PHALCO" recommends varying degrees of exercise with specified FITT parameters based on the BC patient's comorbidities and physical state. We might be able to specify even more precisely which exercise is best for each patient by using this framework as a basis for future therapeutical techniques depending on patient characteristics. Combined training appears to be the best APA strategy able to supplement the conventional therapy, as it has been demonstrated to improve QoL (quality of life), functional ability, muscular strength, and reduce the impression of tiredness. In conclusion, it needs to be incorporated into the BC patient's rehabilitation process from the beginning [26].

4.5 Patients with type 2 diabetes

Globally, type 2 diabetes is a significant public health issue. Even though physical activity (PA) has been shown to have positive benefits on type 2 diabetic patients, a 2009 World Health Organization (WHO) study states that 27% of the disease is caused by physical inactivity [30, 31]. To assist reduce risk factors and avoid metabolic diseases, the French National Health Authority has promoted PA since 2011 by including it as a non-medicinal therapy and an essential component of the type 2 diabetes care route. As per the "Health System Modernization" regulation passed in France in 2016, General Practitioners (GPs) are authorized to recommend adapted physical activity (APA) to patients with long-term illness (LTD) as part of their treatment plan.

The ability to prescribe APA is also granted to paramedical health professionals, such as masseur-physiotherapists, occupational therapists, and psychomotor therapists, as well as health professionals who have completed an Adapted Physical Activity Teachers (APAT) program. In order to lessen the risk factors and functional restrictions associated with his chronic illness, the intervener's job is to help the patient gradually transition to a regular, physically active lifestyle in a safe and customized way. Patient empowerment regarding PA practice is the aim.

The main healthcare providers that are most involved in the management of type 2 diabetes are general practitioners (GPs). For diabetic patients, physical activity (PA) seems to be an essential non-pharmacological treatment in addition to a well-balanced diet. Doctors highlight a few barriers to prescribing it, though. Evaluation of the procedures, obstacles, and elements supporting French Guiana general practitioners' prescription of PA to patients with type 2 diabetes was the goal of the Dranebois et al.'s cross-sectional descriptive survey (2022).

Improving general practitioners' training in the domain of prescribing physical exercise, developing therapeutic education—especially for paramedical staff—and fostering collaboration among various healthcare providers all seem to be crucial. A significant benefit in the treatment of type 2 diabetes would be the creation of sport-health organizations linking sports educators and caregiver's aides. Health insurance may employ financial incentives to encourage physical activity, but in the spirit of health promotion, local governments should provide their citizens with the necessary infrastructures to maintain or improve their health through sports. This is a challenging goal to accomplish in an area where a significant infrastructure gap is caused by rapid population growth and unplanned city expansion. Conclusively, in order to effectively treat type 2 diabetes in French Guiana, it is imperative that general practitioners have better training in prescribing PA, that appropriate PA structures be developed, and that stakeholders in the sport-health system cooperate together [30, 31].

5. Effects of sports on prescription project on patient health and well-being

Programs that promote physical exercise have been shown to have positive benefits in preventing disease progression and primary prevention. A more integrated and multisectoral primary care healthcare delivery system is called for by the French national healthcare policy, "Ma Santé 2022," with a larger emphasis on primary and secondary preventive programs including physical exercise and health education [32]. Since 2012, Sport Santé sur Ordonnance (SSSO), a physical activity program, has been supported by the city of Strasbourg through its Local Health Contracts (CLS), allowing local physicians to prescribe physical exercise to their patients. The three-year physical activity program, which includes individual monitoring (motivational counseling and physical activity assessments), regular sport sessions (adapted physical activity in groups), and sport sessions before to or following a clinical rehabilitation phase, is available to eligible patients without delay. Approximately 4000 people (mean age = 52 years old) were enrolled in these programs at this point [32].

This study was funded by EU through the JADECARE project and examined the functional status, well-being, and impact on healthcare service consumption of patients enrolled in the SSSO program between January 1, 2020, and December 31, 2021 (N = 864; 72% of female and 28% of male participants; 88% of patients have at least one chronic condition, and 28% have at least two). It was unknown how the use of health services may develop in the future. Information was gathered from the SSSO program participant database and cross-referenced with information from the public health insurer (CPAM du Bas Rhin). The patients' functional condition was assessed at the beginning, middle, and end of the program. The utilization of health-care services was compared between program participants' health insurance data and matched non-participants' data. There was matching in terms of diagnosis, age, gender, and location of residence.

Both the physical evaluation and the patient's impression indicated a significant improvement in patients' functional status, according to the research. The well-being score showed a notable improvement. Comparing SSSO service users to non-users, the study of health insurance data revealed some implications on healthcare expenditures, primarily in terms of the frequency of doctor visits and medication usage. It was not possible to demonstrate the benefits across the full intervention period, though, because health insurance data were only available for the first 2 years [32].

The current study suggests that empowering patients and those who are at risk to actively participate in their own health beyond what can be accomplished by medical therapies may benefit patients' functional status and well-being as well as the state of the economy. Rather, it requires linking many databases to identify longitudinal patient data linked to concrete actions. The results' significance may be limited as the current study used rather simplistic methods to match SSSO service users with non-users.

The goal of a related study was to prescribe adaptive physical exercise based on the expectations of patients visiting general practitioners in the Yvelines department in Northern France [33]. Adapted physical activity (APA) has been prescribed by general practitioners to individuals with long-term health issues in France since 2016. In nine doctor's offices, 252 patients completed surveys. 95.2% of patients believe that prescribing APA is a good concept, 80.2% of patients were inspired to enroll in an APA program, and 67.4% of patients believed that prescribing APA would boost their motivation. The biggest barriers to engaging in physical activity were a lack of time (59.9%) and motivation (31.7%). Professional group meetings (64.7%) and follow-up visits with physicians (41.7%) were the main tactics that would help patients adhere to an APA program more successfully. About 53.2% of patients stated that using a connected device to monitor their exercise would be essential. In summary, the findings demonstrated a positive attitude among patients toward APA prescription, which is noteworthy for the promotion of PA in general care [33].

6. Movements and alliances to promote physical activity as medicine

6.1 The "exercise is medicine®" Movement

The "Exercise is Medicine® Health Care Providers' Action Guide" includes easy and practical methods for incorporating physical activity into everyday practice. More than 40 of the most prevalent chronic health disorders may be prevented, treated, and managed for your patients by encouraging the appropriate "dosage" of physical exercise. The global health initiative "Exercise is Medicine" exists in 37 countries worldwide. This initiative aims to promote physical activity and exercise as a treatment for the prevention and treatment of diseases. The countries participating in the initiative are as follows: Argentina, Australia, Austria, Belgium, Brazil, Canada, Chile, China, Colombia, Cyprus, Denmark, Finland, France, Germany.

Hellas, India, Indonesia, Ireland, Israel, Italy, Japan, Latvia, Mexico, Netherlands, New Zealand, Norway, Peru, Philippines, Poland, Portugal, Russia, Singapore, South Africa, Spain, Sweden, Switzerland, and United Kingdom [34].

The prescription of physical exercise by doctors is a practice that has been implemented in various countries. The Central Health Council (KESY) of Greece has approved the workout recommendation, and it is currently being implemented. Training sessions on exercise prescription are offered by the National Center "Exercise is Medicine-Greece." Additionally, some European nations, including France, as well as the United States, Canada, Sweden, England, and Scotland, have adopted the practice of prescribing exercise. The European Federation of Sports Medicine Associations (EFSMA) has provided information. The European Federation of Sports Medicine Associations (EFSMA) established exercise prescription for health to encourage physical activity as a way of illness prevention and treatment. These countries recognize the significant health benefits of physical activity and have integrated it into their healthcare systems.

For more than 20 years, physical exercise prescriptions have been part of healthcare for the first time in Sweden, for instance. Physical Activity on Prescription (PAP-S) is an approach that combines tailored counseling with diagnosis-specific physical activity guidelines. Physical activity can be prescribed by any qualified healthcare provider with the necessary experience. The Public Health Agency of Sweden coordinates an EU-funded project to support the implementation of this method in nine other European countries (Malta, Italy, Flemish, Portugal, Denmark, Germany, Catalonia-Spain, Lithuania, and Romania). For more detailed information, you may want to refer to the Europe Physical Activity Factsheet 2021.

The ultimate goals are to promote good health and avoid noncommunicable diseases by establishing country-based physical activity on prescription (PAP) programs in healthcare systems across various nations [35].

6.2 Exercise guidelines for health and home-based rehabilitation regarding physical activity

Despite being published for over 30 years, several prospective cohort studies on the benefits of regular physical activity have received little attention. However, Loellgen et al.'s research [36] has revealed evidence-based health advantages of exercise. Over a million subjects participate in activities for prevention, treatment, and rehabilitation. Sedentary lifestyle, including lack of exercise, excessive sitting and screen time, and smoking, is a major risk factor for numerous illnesses. After recovering from serious illnesses or being released from hospitals, people require rehabilitation as either inpatients at rehabilitation clinics or as outpatients in ambulant training groups or training facilities. Motivating patients to participate in an intense home-based rehabilitation program under the guidance of a certified training instructor is the main responsibility of a general practitioner. Rehabilitation and exercise training improves overall health, quality of life, physical performance, and longevity. Regular physical exercise is essential for both prevention and recovery. Physical exercise has a range of effects on numerous organs and their functioning. **Figure 2** shows some of the good consequences of frequent physical activity.

Long-term training typically leads to perceived improvements in activities in daily life (ADL) performance. Improved quality of life motivates patients to continue exercising on a regular basis.

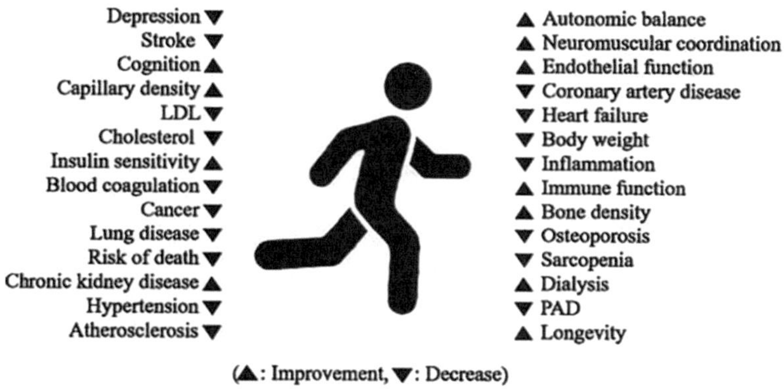

Figure 2.
Some of the good consequences of frequent physical activity [36].

The EFSMA prepared and distributed eighteen tables, which may be found at [37]. Training suggestions that are unique to everyone may be made using the sets of variables included in these tables. It is essential to create a formula that simplifies the many criteria and accounts for age, sickness risk, anthropometric data, and pre-participation test results. A fundamental stage in the intervention process to increase the desire for physical activity appears in **Table 1** as a recommendation for exercise prescription for health (EPH).

Exercise prescription for health (EPH) is a cost-effective method for motivating patients to engage in regular activity and stick to it for extended periods of time (**Figure 3**).

The European sports physicians' guidelines for children's and adults' physical activity.	
Children	• Engage in at least 60 minutes of moderate or strenuous physical exercise every day, including endurance, flexibility, balance, and muscular endurance training at least once.
Adults aged 18 to 65 years	• Aim for 150 minutes of moderate-intensity aerobic activity each week, 75 minutes of vigorous-intensity activity, or a mix of both.
Adults aged 65 years and above	• Aim for at least 150 minutes of moderate-intensity aerobic physical exercise each week, including at least 30 minutes on 5 days and 50 minutes on 3 days. • 75 minutes a week of high-intensity aerobic exercise spread out throughout the week, or a similar mix of moderate-to-high-intensity exercise and moderate-to-intense strength training at least twice a week, along with muscular endurance, flexibility, and balance training. • Aerobic activity can be done at intervals of at least 10 minutes.
Elderly adults with poor mobility	• Exercise to improve equilibrium avoiding falls for three or more days a week. • On at least 2 days each week, engage in muscle-strengthening exercises that target main muscle groups. • Remark: older persons should engage in as much physical exercise as their skills and conditions permit, even if they are unable to meet the recommended daily intake owing to health issues. Resistance exercise refers to physical activity when the patient works against resistance, such as weight.
Adapted from: Loellgen [36].	

Table 1.
The physical activity prescription for health (EPH).

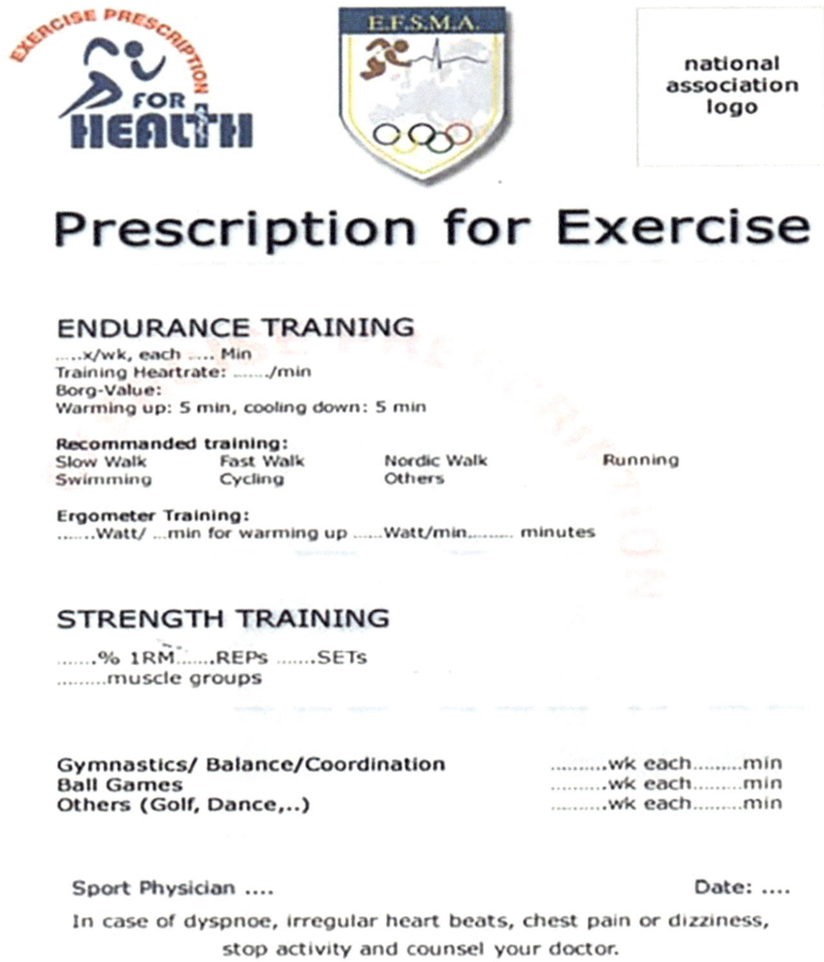
national association logo

Prescription for Exercise

ENDURANCE TRAINING
.....x/wk, each ..... Min
Training Heartrate: ..../min
Borg-Value:
Warming up: 5 min, cooling down: 5 min

Recommanded training:

Slow Walk	Fast Walk	Nordic Walk	Running
Swimming	Cycling	Others	

Ergometer Training:
.......Watt/ ...min for warming up ......Watt/min......... minutes

STRENGTH TRAINING
.......% 1RM.......REPs ....SETs
.........muscle groups

Gymnastics/ Balance/Coordination	..........wk each.........min
Ball Games	..........wk each.........min
Others (Golf, Dance,..)	..........wk each.........min

Sport Physician .... Date: ....

In case of dyspnoe, irregular heart beats, chest pain or dizziness, stop activity and counsel your doctor.

Figure 3.
The example of the recipe for the exercise prescription for health (see [36, 37]: www.efsma.eu).

6.3 The Hamburg declaration: an international alliance to promote physical activity

As a result of decreased PA, obesity is becoming a global epidemic. Children are impacted, as are all age groups. Insufficient PA leads to a great deal of issues for both people and society. Blood diseases, diabetes, heart disease, depression, and the uncontrollably rising demand on our health systems are all contributing factors, as are growing infrastructure costs and millions of dollars in lost productivity due to people's inability to work. The solution is to encourage more individuals to move. This is the main objective of the "Global Alliance for the Promotion of Physical Activity," which is backed by more than 139 organizations globally, including the IOC, and is spelled out in the Hamburg Declaration [38]. The main objective is to get individuals moving, regardless of their own baseline level, as a means of increasing physical activity and participation in sports. Achieving this goal will enhance people's quality of life, save lives, save money, and promote world peace. These are the five key messages that the GA is promoting:

a. Promote physical activity as a kind of medicine. To spread the word that happiness, health, and well-being start at home, use role models and influencers in all facets of your life. PA is the most effective medication. Prevention is more effective than treatment.

b. Influencing those who make decisions. Develop tools and methods for GA members to persuade governments, corporations, and nongovernmental organizations to invest in PA to save lives, save money, and benefit society.

c. Adapting physical activity to individuals, communities, and environment. Individualized physical activity should take into account age, gender, socioeconomic status, cultural background, and climate conditions [39].

d. Make use of modern technology. Collaborate with major tech firms, pharmaceutical and healthcare organizations, and academic institutions to integrate wearable technology, cell phones, the Internet, and the metaverse into everyday life. To make it easy and fun for people to join PA, you can use gamification, incentives, and community growth.

e. A request for additional policy and program efficacy trials. Most knowledge on prevention comes from cohort studies. However, well-designed trials of physical exercise in communities and the healthcare system are urgently required, particularly for underserved minorities.

Licensed healthcare professionals in Swedish primary care, including physicians, physiotherapists, and nurses, can prescribe PA if they are trained in patient-centered counseling and the FaR method, as well as knowledge of the patient's current state of health. Patients in primary care have higher levels of PA after 6 and 12 months of using the FaR technique in clinical settings. Fysisk aktivitet på recept (FaR), in English means 'Physical activity on prescription' (PAP-S) [40]. Implementation tools and delivery mechanisms must be easily accessible in order to reduce obstacles. Pedometer usage, the FaR method, and handbooks like FYSS are a few examples. The written prescription that results from the counseling is based on the FYSS guidebook [38].

Individual physical activity is preferred by many patients. It is said that walking is the most favored physical exercise. Pedometers are a frequent tool used by Swedish physiotherapists in response to the Swedish Council on Technology Assessment in Health Care (SBU) report to encourage greater levels of physical activity. The follow-up, which involves tracking improvement and even modifying the prescription, is crucial. It is feasible to close the gap between research and practice using a verified pedometer. The FaR system in Swedish used evidence-based strategies to promote physical activity and found that pedometer-based physical activity intervention programs had the biggest impact size [41].

The way PAP-S's five essential components interact is what makes it special. Individualized written prescriptions with follow-ups are produced by person-centered counseling that incorporates evidence-based, diagnosis-specific physical activity recommendations. Furthermore, healthcare providers work with local

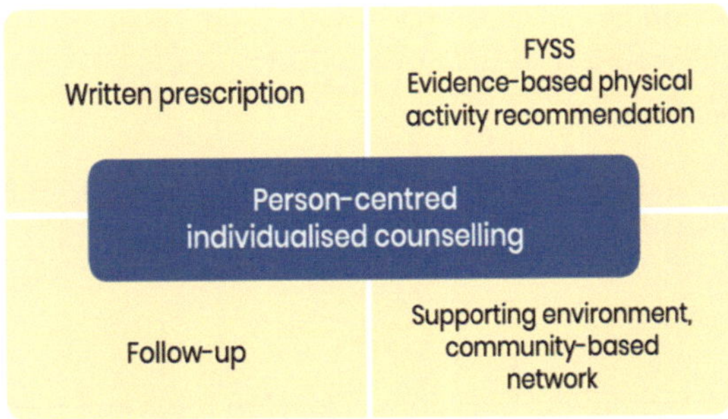

Figure 4.
The PAP-S approach consists of five key components [40].

activity organizers to assist people improve and maintain their level of exercise [41, 42]. *"An advantage of PAP-S in Sweden is that all licensed health professionals, with adequate expertise, can prescribe physical activity, not only doctors" (Physical Activity in the Prevention and Treatment of Disease, FYSS)* (**Figure 4**).

7. Authority and barriers in adaptive exercise prescription

7.1 Primary care doctors'

The "exercise pill" has never been more consistently recommended by scientific evidence and international standards for a wide range of chronic diseases, emphasizing the necessity of customizing the prescription to the patient's circumstances (much as with pharmacological prescriptions). But does medicine actually recommend physical activity? Are medical professionals qualified to recommend exercise? Do fitness experts possess specialized knowledge about modifying exercise for those with long-term medical conditions? [43].

Based on current statistics, it appears that doctors still seldom prescribe structured, individual physical activity, and there is a significant cultural difference in the training that separates doctors from other healthcare providers [44]. Lack of a wide geographical network of facilities appropriate for the application of physical exercise programs as medical treatments for the primary chronic and noncommunicable illnesses makes a successful implementation even more difficult.

Based on these presumptions, the study by Battista et al. [43] examined the effects of a Massive Open Online Course (MOOC) on the functional assessment, recommendation, and usage of individually tailored physical exercise in medicine. This particular kind of instruction aims to close the gap between clinical settings and gyms by offering unique, cutting-edge, and engaging higher education tactics. "Exercise in Medicine: From Functional Evaluation to Adapted Exercise Training" is an MOOC that is made available to the public worldwide as an open-access educational resource by the Sports and Exercise Medicine Division of the Department of Medicine at the University of Padova (Italy).

Experts from across the world may share their thoughts and ideas through the e-learning platform Future Learn, which is facilitated by qualified educators. Additionally, this interactive MOOC can help worldwide projects focusing on exercise in medicine creating a network.

The ultimate goal of the MOOC is to teach participants how to include exercise as a medical treatment into healthcare systems and how to use functional evaluation for adapted exercise prescription. MOOC is a suitable educational method for physicians' training. Worldwide, there is currently a deficiency in training about functional evaluation and prescription of exercises. The primary obstacle to prescribing and implementing exercise in everyday practice, according to several healthcare and fitness experts, is an ability gap that must be filled via training.

Given the excellent user satisfaction ratings that the MOOC has garnered, it appears that professionals with an interest in the subject matter find that the autonomous learner-centered training modalities and communication facilitate their ability to meet their requirements and accomplish the learning objectives [43].

To create a society that is healthier and more physically active in the future, healthcare and fitness experts, as well as the general public, need to start by sharing instructional materials and projects. For these strong reasons, policymakers and all major medical higher education institutions should have customized exercise prescription as a shared goal.

The authors suggested that fundamentals and advantages of a physically active and healthy lifestyle should be promoted among the public, and all health professionals should possess at least a basic understanding of how to prescribe and implement individualized exercise programs. In the constraints of their own surroundings, everyone will be able to contribute to the creation of a more active and hence healthier world in this way (**Figure 5**) [43].

Considerable new information was obtained from Tchirkov et al.'s meta-analytic study [46], which examined the challenges that doctors, and their patients continue to face, and which impede the usefulness and accessibility of adapted physical activity (APA). About 22 French medical theses between 2016 and 2020 were included in this

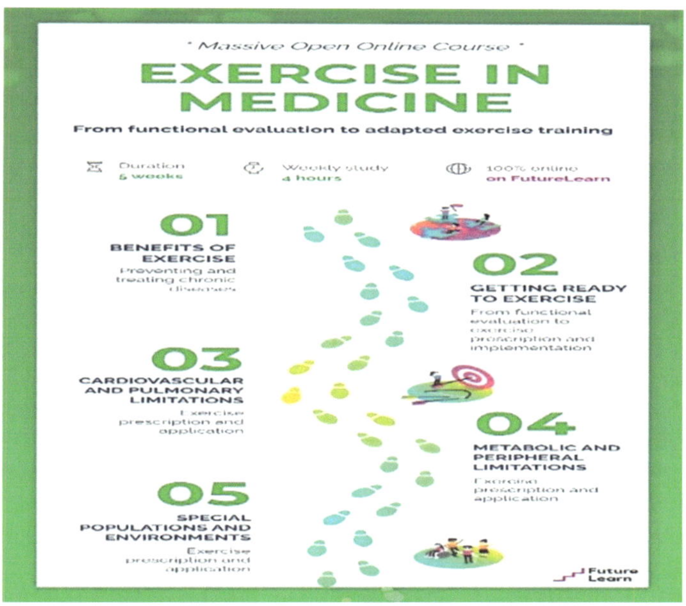
" Massive Open Online Course "
EXERCISE IN MEDICINE
From functional evaluation to adapted exercise training
Duration
5 weeks
Weekly study
4 hours
100% online
on FutureLearn
01
BENEFITS OF EXERCISE
Preventing and treating chronic
02
GETTING READY TO EXERCISE
From functional evaluation to
prescription and implementation
03
CARDIOVASCULAR AND PULMONARY LIMITATIONS
Exercise prescription and application
04
METABOLIC AND PERIPHERAL LIMITATIONS
prescription and application
05
SPECIAL POPULATIONS AND ENVIRONMENTS
Exercise
Future Learn

Figure 5.
A diagram that summarizes the subjects covered in each course week. See the weekly summary of each week's theme content may be viewed by clicking on [45].

meta-analysis. According to this study, General Practitioners (GPs) in France are now able to recommend APA to patients who have a long-term disease as a result of recent legislation aimed at modernizing the healthcare system (the 2016 French Healthcare Act and its Implementing Decree). The results showed that, during the time period under investigation, relatively few general practitioners prescribed APA in spite of the new laws. Insufficient time during consultations, inadequate training, uncertainty regarding patient referrals for APA, and skepticism toward APA practitioners seemed to be the primary barriers to APA prescription as a nonpharmacological treatment. The choice to prescribe APA appeared to be influenced by the GP's lifestyle, the nature of the patient-physician connection, and the GP's assessment of the patient's attitude toward sports. Neither the scientific literature nor the most current regulations pertaining to the introduction of APA prescription in France have given much consideration to the perspective of general practitioners (physicians). The results of this meta-analysis indicate that further study and legislation are required, with a focus on taking into account the viewpoints of prescribing doctors and their interactions with patients.

The data in the single-case studies that were taken from the theses, which were frequently characterized by poor statistical significance and based on very small and unrepresentative samples, should be the first consideration when assessing the representativeness of the data in the present meta-analysis. Another theory is that the general practitioners who consented to take part in the research listed above were the ones who were most in favor of the APA's prescription. Therefore, less weight was given to the opinions of general practitioners who disagreed with APA prescriptions. Between the interviewers, who were interns, and their interviewees, general practitioners who frequently oversaw interns, there was also a certain level of familiarity or respect [46].

The single-case studies that were taken from the theses, which were frequently characterized by poor statistical significance and based on very small and unrepresentative samples, were the first of the meta-analysis' shortcomings. Additionally, there was a certain level of familiarity or deference between the interviewees (GPs who frequently oversaw interns) and the interviewers (interns). This meta-analysis was based on 22 internist medical theses that examined general practitioners' opinions on APA. A lot of quantitative data revealed distinct patterns and provide a current summary of APA prescription practices in France.

Tchirkov et al.'s [47] literature review on the use of adapted physical exercise to treat chronic illness examined barriers to prescription. As physical exercise has been linked to so many health advantages, especially for chronic diseases, it is now recognized as a stand-alone therapy. Nonetheless, general practitioners continue to prescribe physical exercise infrequently and face many challenges. This study of the literature aims to pinpoint these challenges for doctors and patients with chronic illnesses, specifically in France. The literature evaluation was based on 44 relevant publications that were kept from peer-reviewed journals, medical theses, and public health reports that were published in either French or English between 2000 and 2020.

The biggest barriers for doctors to recommend adapted physical activity were time constraints during consultations, a lack of training, and ignorance of adapted physical activity or where to direct patients. Other barriers were the nature of the relationship between the physician and the patient or the personal habits and views of the doctors about physical exercise. Patients' obstacles included not having enough time or desire, limited access to "sport for health" programs, and cultural distancing from physical activity. Noncompliance was found to be correlated with age, educational attainment, or socio-professional category.

The findings pointed to many directions for raising prescription rates and enhancing compliance with adapted physical activity. Enhancing medical education in this area, creating guidelines to make prescription processes easier, assessing patients' physical and psychological states, and reducing socioeconomic disparities that affect people's access to health services and physical exercise are a few examples. In order to mainstream health standards and accomplish public health goals, the main goal of "sport for health" programs is "to convert the person's lifestyle into a physically active one" [48]. There are still numerous challenges in the way of efforts to enhance the health of individuals with chronic illnesses and encourage adaptive physical exercise. Neither patient expectations nor medical training nor practices have yet to firmly establish the recommendation for adapted physical activity.

The descriptive Survey of General Practitioners in Prescription Physical Activity: Case of Khouribga Province, Morocco, revealed similar results [49]. The study was conducted in 2021 between April and June to assess the general practitioners' (GPs') understanding of prescribing adapted physical activity (APA), as well as their viewpoints, experiences, feelings, and barriers to doing so (PA). According to the findings, 92% of general practitioners advised patients to get APAs. Just 6.41% of the physicians provided quantifiable goals to be met (the amount of time and frequency of physical exercise), and none of them said they provided a comprehensive program that specified the kind, level of intensity, frequency, and length of each session. Prescriptions from the APA were practically 100% oral.

The least common approach was the written prescription, while 30.58% of respondents gave a PA information leaflet. Both autonomy and quality of life are intended to be preserved by the planned APAs. The patients' lack of enthusiasm, lack of time, and ignorance of the subject matter were the biggest obstacles to the prescription. Both the quantity and effectiveness of medical prescriptions for APA would surely be enhanced by better knowledge on APA prescription procedures and the frameworks that provide collaboration with sports medicine services and sports medicine educators [49].

7.2 Toolkit for fitness trainers and instructors

Important research [50] aimed to improve knowledge, skills, and self-efficacy among Adaptavie workers. After conducting focus groups and reviewing research, Adaptavie's kinesiologists collaborated to develop an APA toolkit to meet this requirement. The APA toolkit demonstrated great usability and integrity, leading to increased knowledge and self-efficacy in the workplace. Kinesiologists reported that the toolkit improved knowledge, abilities, and confidence in accessing credible APA resources, leading to a substantial improvement in job self-efficacy after 1 year of use. Given that the toolkit's prescriptions are supported by empirical data, kinesiologists who utilize it to prescribe APA may find that their clients with impairments benefit more from it. Personalized physical exercise programs have been linked to increased involvement, motivation, personal growth, and self-efficacy. The toolkit's availability in both paper and electronic versions, as well as in French and English, should aid in its adoption and possible application in the field [50].

This study has limitations due to the limited sample size of kinesiologists from a single community group. Other health professionals that offer APA services include coaches, physical education experts, occupational therapists, and physiotherapists; these professionals were left out of this study. Furthermore, throughout the research period, there were personnel changes, and kinesiologists' availability varied (e.g., through part-time work or a severe workload). As a result, there was variation among responders throughout the research.

Adaptavie highlighted the need for an evidence-based toolbox to promote knowledge and self-efficacy in delivering APA services for individuals with disabilities. The toolbox boosted self-efficacy in the workplace, and all participants found it useful. The future plan includes expanding the toolkit to additional community groups with comparable needs and incorporating it into the Quebec university curriculum for kinesiologists, where APA training is currently lacking [50].

8. Conclusion

The global project "exercise prescription for health and disease prevention" has its roots in antiquity, almost two millennia ago. Hippocrates of Greece was the first "recorded" physician to write an exercise prescription for a patient suffering from consumption, and Galen of Rome's guidance on the use of exercise for patients in illness treatment remained influential until the sixteenth century. Exercise has historically been linked to diabetes, obesity, and inactivity as some medical practitioners have recommended it to reduce these health concerns. For both the body and the mind, "Exercise is Medicine" is among the most important healthcare concerns of the twenty-first century. Exercise is a modifiable lifestyle component as research has shown that it has a positive impact on holistic human performance across the lifetime. The lack of training appears to be the most significant barrier to the universality of PA prescription. Training organization and the development of particular tools for attending physicians appear to be interesting alternatives. The fourth most common cause of mortality worldwide is physical inactivity. Physical activity (PA) prescriptions by doctors are now outlined in legislation that emphasizes the primary role of family physicians. It is needed to be done more research on general practitioners' (GPs') needs regarding prescribing PA. It is proposed that enhancing individual motivation and ability in addition to using a systems approach (socio-ecological model) is necessary for the effective use of PA in healthcare [41].

Policymakers, healthcare leaders, and professional groups should all provide general support. Facilitating the process requires easily accessible implementation tools and delivery systems. Examples include evidence-based guidelines like FYSS and physical activity on prescription systems, as well as strategies like using pedometers. According to Hellenius and Sundberg [51], the FYSS book has been translated into English, Norwegian, and Vietnamese. Talks about translating it into other languages are still in progress. Swedish Professional Associations for Physical Activity actively seek international collaborators for future translations.

It has been proposed that a systems approach (socio-ecological model) and the development of personal motivation and competence are necessary for the successful use of physical activity counseling in healthcare [52]. To begin, legislators, healthcare leaders, and professional associations must all provide their support.

These actions boost motivation by raising awareness and validity.

DOI: http://dx.doi.org/10.5772/intechopen.1004542

Author details

Katerina Asonitou[1,2*], Soteria Yiannaki[2,3*] and Dimitra Koutsouki[1,2]

1 Laboratory of Adapted Physical Activity/Developmental and Physical Disabilities, National and Kapodistrian University of Athens, Greece

2 School of Physical Education and Sport Science, National and Kapodistrian University of Athens, Greece

3 Faculty of History of Physical Education and Sport, National and Kapodistrian University of Athens, Greece

*Address all correspondence to: kasonitou@phed.uoa.gr and sgiannaki@phed.uoa.gr

References

[1] Barbin J, Camy J, Communal DMF, Perrin C, Vergnault M. Référentiel d'activité et de compétences de l'enseignant en activité physique adaptée. 2015. Available from: http://pmbsoie.univlyon1.fr/doc_num.php?explnum_id=512

[2] Thornton JS, Frémont P, Khan K, Poirier P, Fowles J, Wells GD, et al. Physical activity prescription: A critical opportunity to address a modifiable risk factor for the prevention and Management of Chronic Disease: A position statement by the Canadian academy of sport and exercise medicine. Clinical Journal of Sport Medicine. 2016;**26**(4):259-265. DOI: 10.1097/JSM.0000000000000363

[3] Harvard-School of Public Health [Internet]. 2023. Available from: https://www.hsph.harvard.edu/nutritionsource/physical-activity-considerations-special-populations/

[4] JADECARE insights in original Good Practice transfer: Effects of 'Sports on Prescription' on Patient Health and Wellbeing. 2023. Available from: https://www.jadecare.eu/jadecare-insights-in-original-good-practice-transfer-effects-of-sports-on-prescription-on-patient-health-and-wellbeing/

[5] Plato, Theaetetus 153a-c

[6] Tipton CM. Historical perspective: The antiquity of exercise, exercise physiology and the exercise prescription for health. World Review of Nutrition and Dietetics. 2008;**98**:198-245. DOI: 0.1159/000152989

[7] Homeric Hymns 16

[8] Hippocrates, Regimen 2.25-28; Aphorismi 1.3; Epidemics 6.4.18.3

[9] Kleisiaris CF, Sfakianakis C, Papathanasiou IV. Health care practices in ancient Greece: The Hippocratic ideal. Journal of Medical Ethics and History of Medicine. 2014;7:6

[10] Plato, Laws 2.673a; Plato Republic 2.376e; Plato, Republic 3.411d; Plato Laws 7.795d; Plato, Republic 3.403c-d; Plato, Gorgias 464b; Plato, Protagoras 326b-c; Plato, Timaeus, 88b-c

[11] Plato, Timaeus 87d; Plato, Timaeus 88b; Plato, Republic 3.403c-d

[12] Aristotle, Politics 7.1332a; Aristotle, Politics 7.1331b-1332a; Aristotle, Nicomachean Ethics 1096b; Aristotle, Politics 7.1335b; Aristotle, Nicomachean Ethics, 1104a

[13] Pavlogiannis O, Lomi C, Albanidis E, Konitsiotis S, Geroulanos S. Sport and medicine during Greek antiquity and roman imperial times. Journal of the Washington Academy of Sciences. 2007;**93**(1):59-75. Available from: http://www.jstor.org/stable/24536252

[14] Plutarch, De liberis educanids 10.; Plutarch, De liberis educanids 9

[15] Galen, De sanitate tuenda libri VI.85; Galen, Thrasybulus IX 820; Galen, Thrasybulus XXVIII 858; Galen, Thrasybulus IV 811-813; Galen, Thrasybulus XXXV 872-873

[16] Philostratos, Gymnastikos 14

[17] Plato, Republic 3.406a-b; Plato, Crito 47b; Plato, Gorgias 504a; Plato, Gorgias 464a; Plato, Sophist 227a; Plato, Protagoras 313d

[18] Yiannakis T. History of Physical Education (in Greek). Athens: Self-published; 1998. pp. 17-20

[19] Berryman JW. Exercise is medicine: A historical perspective. Current Sports Medicine Reports. 2010;**9**(4):195-201. DOI: 10.1249/JSR.0b013e3181e7d86d

[20] Joelsson M, Lundqvist S, Larsson MEH. Tailored physical activity on prescription with follow-ups improved motivation and physical activity levels. A qualitative study of a 5-year Swedish primary care intervention. Scandinavian Journal of Primary Health Care. 2020;**38**(4):399-410. DOI: 10.1080/02813432.2020.1842965

[21] Pedersen BK, Saltin B. Exercise as medicine - evidence for prescribing exercise as therapy in 26 different chronic diseases. Scandinavian Journal of Medicine & Science in Sports. 2015;**25**(Suppl. 3):1-72. DOI: 10.1111/sms.12581

[22] Allado E, Poussel M, Albuisson E, Paysant J, Temperelli M, Hily O, et al. Real intensity of physical activity capacity of patients with chronic disease: A cross-sectional study. Scientific Reports. 2022;**12**(1):12593. DOI: 10.1038/s41598-022-17047-9

[23] Clanchy KM, Tweedy SM, Trost SG. The adapted physical activity program: A theory-driven, evidence-based physical activity intervention for people with brain impairment. Brain Impairment. 2019;**20**(1):81-95. DOI: 10.1017/BrImp.2018.16

[24] Asonitou K, Mpampoulis T, Irakleous-Paleologou H, Koutsouki D. Effects of an adapted physical activity program on physical fitness of adults with intellectual disabilities. Advances in Physical Education. 2018;**8**:321-336. DOI: 10.4236/ape.2018.83028

[25] Bernhardsson S, Boman C, Lundqvist S, et al. Implementation of physical activity on prescription for children with obesity in pediatric health care (IMPA): Protocol for a feasibility and evaluation study using quantitative and qualitative methods. Pilot and Feasibility Studies. 2022;**8**:117. DOI: 10.1186/s40814-022-01075-3

[26] Murri A, Vitucci D, Tranchita E, Grazioli E, Gori S, Modena A, et al. "OPERATION PHALCO"—Adapted physical activity for breast cancer survivors: Is it time for a multidisciplinary approach? Cancers. 2023;**15**:34. DOI: 10.3390/cancers15010034

[27] Schutz S, Aidar FJ. Different methods of physical training applied to women breast cancer survivors: A systematic review. Frontiers in Physiology. 2021;**12**:639406

[28] Natalucci V, Villarini M, Emili R, Acito M, Vallorani L, Barbieri E, et al. Special attention to physical activity in breast cancer patients during the first wave of COVID-19 pandemic in Italy: The Diana web cohort. Journal of Personalized Medicine. 2021;**11**:381

[29] Galiano-Castillo N, Arroyo-Morales M. The six-minute walk test as a measure of health in breast cancer patients. Journal of Aging and Physical Activity. 2016;**24**:508-515

[30] Millor N, Lecumberri P. An evaluation of the 30-s chair stand test in older adults: Frailty detection based on kinematic parameters from a single inertial unit. Journal of Neuroengineering and Rehabilitation. 2013;**10**:86

[31] Dranebois S, Lalanne-Mistrih ML, Nacher M, Thelusme L, Deungoue S, Demar M, et al. Prescription of physical activity by general practitioners in type 2 diabetes: Practice and barriers in French Guiana. Frontiers in Endocrinology.

2022;**12**:790326. DOI: 10.3389/fendo.2021.790326

[32] Schuster C et al. Effects of a sports on prescription project on patient health and wellbeing. International Journal of Integrated Care. 2022;**22**(S3):249. DOI: doi.org/10.5334/ijic.ICIC22249

[33] Kanso C, Blanchard J-C, Astruc A. P07-02 prescription of adapted physical activity: Expectations of patients consulting general practitioners in the department of Yvelines. European Journal of Public Health. 2022;**32**(Sup plement_2):ckac095.102. DOI: 10.1093/eurpub/ckac095.102

[34] Exercise is Medicine. Available from: https://www.exerciseismedicine.org/eim_map/

[35] An effective model to increase physical activity. Available from: https://www.eupap.org/

[36] Loellgen H, Zupet P, Bachl N, Debruyne A. Physical activity, exercise prescription for health and home-based rehabilitation. Sustainability. 2020;**12**(24):10230. DOI: 10.3390/su122410230

[37] European Federation of Sports Medicine Associations. Available from: www.efsma.eu

[38] Andersen P, Holmberg S, Årestedt K. et al. Factors associated with increased physical activity among patients prescribed physical activity in Swedish routine health care including an offer of counselor support: A 1-year follow-up. BMC Public Health. 2022;**22**:509. DOI: 10.1186/s12889-022-12940-4

[39] Heath GW, Parra DC, Sarmiento OL, Andersen LB, Owen N, Goenka S, et al. Lancet physical activity series working group. Evidence-based intervention in physical activity: Lessons from around the world. Lancet. 2012;**380**(9838):272-281. DOI: 10.1016/S0140-6736(12)60816-2

[40] 20 years of Swedish experience with prescribed physical exercise. Available from: https://eurohealthnet-magazine.eu/physical-activity-on-prescription-exporting-20-years-of-swedish-experience/

[41] Raustorp A, Sundberg CJ. The evolution of physical activity on prescription (FaR) in Sweden. Schweizerische Zeitschrift für Sportmedizin und Sporttraumatologie. 2014;**62**(2):23-25. DOI: 10.34045/SSEM/2014/10

[42] Lundqvist EB, Björk MP, Bernhardsson S. Physical activity on prescription in Swedish primary care: A survey on use, views, and implementation determinants amongst general practitioners. Scandinavian Journal of Primary Health Care. 2024;**42**(1):61-71. DOI: 10.1080/02813432.2023.2288126

[43] Battista F, Sarri C, Foccardi G, Quinto G, Faggian S, Vecchiato M, et al. "Exercise in medicine: From functional evaluation to adapted exercise training": A massive open online course to respond to the burning need for exercise prescription to combat chronic diseases. Deutsche Zeitschrift für Sportmedizin. 2023;**74**:193-196. DOI: 10.5960/dzsm.2023.574

[44] Foccardi G, Hansen D, Quinto G, Favero C, Coninx K, Ruiz GR, et al. How do general practitioners assess physical activity and prescribe exercise in patients with different cardiovascular diseases? An Italian pilot study. European Journal of Preventive Cardiology. 2021;**28**:e20-e24. DOI: 10.1177/2047487320925221

[45] The weekly summary of each week's theme content in each online course of

MOOC. Available from: https://view.genial.ly/637f8df025d1600011c4c092

[46] Tchirkov V et al. Methods and barriers to the prescription of physical activity to patients with chronic illness: The viewpoint of general practitioners. American Journal of Biomedical Science and Research. 2023;**19**(1):64-70. DOI: 10.34297/AJBSR.2023.19.002551

[47] Tchirkov V, Didierjean R, Schuft L. Adapted physical activity to treat chronic disease: A literature review of obstacles to prescription and compliance. Trends in Medicine. 2021;**21**(3):1-5. DOI: 10.15761/TiM.1000274

[48] Barth N, Perrin C, Camy J. Engaging in regular physical activity when you have type 2 diabetes: Between "disease trajectory" and "adapted physical activity (APA) career". Loisir et Société/ Society and Leisure. 2014;**37**:224-240

[49] Imad FE. Survey of general practitioners in prescribing physical activity: Case of Khouribga Province. Journal of Medicine and Public Health. 2023;**4**(7):1087

[50] de Serres-Lafontaine A, Périnet-Lacroix R, Batcho CS, Best KL. Co-creation and evaluation of an adapted physical activity toolkit: Guidelines to support practice among rehabilitation professionals in community organizations. Physical Activity and Health. 2023;7(1): 166-177. DOI: 10.5334/paah.239

[51] Hellénius ML, Sundberg CJ. Physical activity as medicine – Time to translate evidence into clinical practice (editorial). British Journal of Sports Medicine. 2011;**45**(3):158

[52] Börjesson M, Sundberg CJ. FYSS (physical activity book for prevention and treatment): Behavioural change also for the physician? British Journal of Sports Medicine. 2013;**47**(15):937-938

Chapter 3

Exercise is Medicine

Endang Ernandini and Jonathan Alvin Wiryaputra

Abstract

Moving aerobically means moving using oxygen. Our muscles move by using oxygen as their fuel. In various studies, after 30 minutes of aerobic physical exercise, the concentration of free fatty acids in the blood significantly increases. This indicates that, from the 30-minute mark, fats start to mobilize from adipose tissue. Aerobic exercise and endurance training are highly effective in improving physical performance. Anaerobic is a state in which our body moves without oxygen intake. This state can occur, but only for a short period, ranging up to 14 seconds, after which mitochondria must resume working with oxygen as fuel. Despite short-term aerobic exercise training in IR patients, it has a positive effect as a trigger for needs frequency, intensity, time, and type. Frequency is how many days you do exercise in a week. Intensity is how hard exercise is done based on heart rate calculations. Time is how many hours you do exercise in a week. Type exercise could be aerobic, anaerobic, or muscle strengthening.

Keywords: exercise, medicine, aerobic, anaerobic, endurance

1. Introduction

All activities carried out by humans are movements that represent cooperation from head to toe integrated from the abilities and coordination of the brain, cardio, pulmonary, muscles, ligaments, and even all organs that support life [1–3] from organ-level metabolism to cell-level. All these activities are carried out comprehensively and cannot be compartmentalized. Weakness on one side will become weakness and even cause pain throughout the body [4, 5]. An injury to the elbow is not just a matter of the elbow but of the entire arm, trunk, and even the whole body [6, 7].

In this dynamic system that remains integrated in one order, it will be more harmonious when arranged carefully, studied, researched, and performed, so that it can be agreed that exercise is also a prescription for fitness and even healing, and thus it can be said that exercise is medicine [8–10].

Aerobic means using oxygen. Moving aerobically means moving using oxygen. Our muscles move by using oxygen as their fuel. This movement requires a supply of oxygen pumped and circulated through the bloodstream. The lungs must meet the demand for oxygen as fuel, and we will breathe as quickly as possible to meet that oxygen debt. Our hearts beat rapidly to meet this oxygen demand and deliver it to the cells [11].

The subjective and objective experiences of aerobic exercise can vary from person to person. Subjectively, it can be felt differently by each individual or perhaps felt the same but with different levels or thresholds. Objectively, the workload of aerobic exercise can be measured in simple ways, such as measuring our pulse. More advanced measurements can be obtained from the results of a cardiopulmonary exercise test (CPET) [12].

Anaerobic is a state in which our body moves without oxygen intake. This state can occur, but only for a short period, ranging up to 14 seconds, after which mitochondria must resume working with oxygen as fuel. Do we often engage in anaerobic movements? Yes, of course. In our daily lives, we rarely perform movements in an anaerobic state, but during exercise, anaerobic movements can occur. An example is sprinting 100 meters in sports. Anaerobic movements can be performed at high speeds with high explosive power but in a short time. In everyday life, anaerobic movements can occur when we have to hurry, for example, when urgently trying to reach a destination, such as when chasing someone [11, 13].

How do we know the benefits and drawbacks of exercising? In what conditions can we exercise or engage in sports? To what extent should we do it? The body undergoes various activities from a holistic level, starting from cells to organ levels. The main organs involved are the heart, lungs, and muscles. When engaging in activities, the entire body collaborates to ensure that the goals are achieved [14].

Physical fitness describes a person's ability to sustain daily activities with full energy, awareness, and without excessive fatigue [11]. Physical fitness is evaluated based on the following five components [13]:

1. Cardiorespiratory endurance: the ability of the circulatory and respiratory systems to supply oxygen and nutrients during physical activity.

2. Body composition: the proportion of muscle, fat, and bone.

3. Muscle strength: the maximum force generated by muscles or muscle groups at a specific speed.

4. Muscle endurance: the ability of muscles to perform activities without causing excessive fatigue.

5. Flexibility: the range of joint motion for achieving movements [11, 12].

These components are related to the body's abilities that need to be trained, such as agility, coordination, balance, power, reaction time, and speed.

2. Energy metabolism for physical exercise

Physical activity begins with the contraction of skeletal muscles, involving complex interactions between neural and local regulations [14]. This complex interaction is also strongly influenced by hormones, as hormones play a role in muscle development. Testosterone hormone gives characteristic differences between males and females, as it increases male muscle mass by more than 50% compared to females [15].

The body increases the demand for supplies when physical activity occurs through the mechanisms of delivering oxygen and nutrients as fuel to produce energy. The energy source needed to initiate active processes in moving skeletal muscles, and forming physical activities, is known as adenosine triphosphate (ATP). A small amount of ATP is formed in muscle fibers when contraction begins. Only during this brief period is ATP used for muscle contraction and converted into adenosine diphosphate (ADP).

Another compound, phosphocreatine (PCr), transfers energy from high-energy phosphate bonds to ADP, replenishing the muscle's ATP supply (**Figure 1**) [14, 15].

Energy reserves in muscles can only last for about 15 seconds for heavy physical exercises such as sprinting or weightlifting. After 15 seconds, muscle fibers must form additional ATP from stored energy in nutrition. Some nutrition molecules are stored in muscles, but many must be transferred from the liver and adipose tissues, and then transported through the circulatory system into the muscles [14]. The main sources of energy formation are carbohydrates and fats. If cells have enough oxygen storage for oxidative phosphorylation, glucose and fatty acids can be metabolized to produce and supply ATP. Over time, the energy production obtained from glucose and fatty acids through aerobic pathways decreases, and glucose metabolism automatically switches to anaerobic pathways [14].

The most effective ATP production occurs through the aerobic pathway, such as the glycolysis-citric acid cycle, compared to the anaerobic pathway. This is due to the difference in the amount of ATP produced, namely 32 ATP from the aerobic pathway and 2 ATP from the anaerobic pathway [16]. The aerobic pathway involves cellular respiration, which breaks down energy-rich molecules to produce ATP using oxygen (O2) and generates carbon dioxide (CO_2) in the process. Broadly speaking, aerobic metabolism consists of three main stages: glycolysis, the citric acid cycle, and oxidative phosphorylation. Glycolysis, occurring in the cell's cytosol, converts primary energy sources such as glucose and other molecules into pyruvate, producing 2 ATP. The produced pyruvate is transported to the mitochondria matrix to enter the citric acid cycle, resulting in the next stage with the production of NADH (reduced nicotinamide adenine dinucleotide-NAD) and FADH2 (reduced flavin adenine dinucleotide-FAD), and contributing to an additional 2 ATP. Oxidative phosphorylation, taking place in the inner mitochondrial membrane, can generate 28 ATP through the electron transport system and chemiosmosis [16].

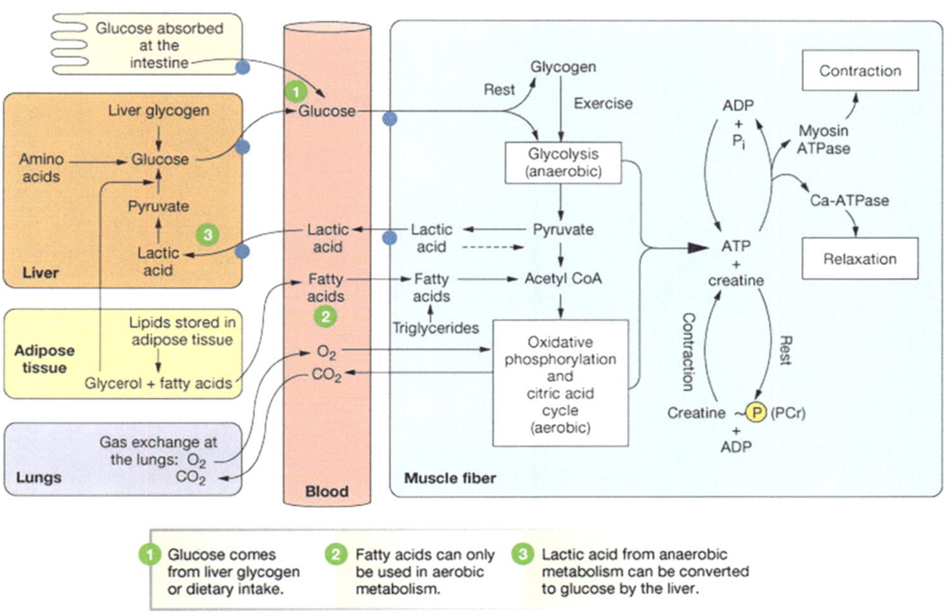

Figure 1.
Cell respiration and ATP production [16].

The anaerobic pathway is characterized by low oxygen levels. When cells lack oxygen for oxidative phosphorylation, the end product of glycolysis, pyruvate, is converted into lactate instead of acetyl-CoA, which would enter the citric acid cycle [14]. Anaerobic metabolism has advantages in terms of early time and speed, as it can metabolize and produce ATP 2.5 times faster than aerobic metabolism. However, this advantage comes with two disadvantages: (a) anaerobic metabolism only produces 2 ATP for every glucose used, while in the aerobic or oxidative process, each processed glucose will yield 30–32 ATP. (b) Anaerobic metabolism contributes to the occurrence of metabolic acidosis by producing H+ (**Figure 2**) [14].

The body has three glucose storage sites: in blood plasma, intracellular muscle, and the liver in the form of glycogen, as well as newly produced glucose by the liver through

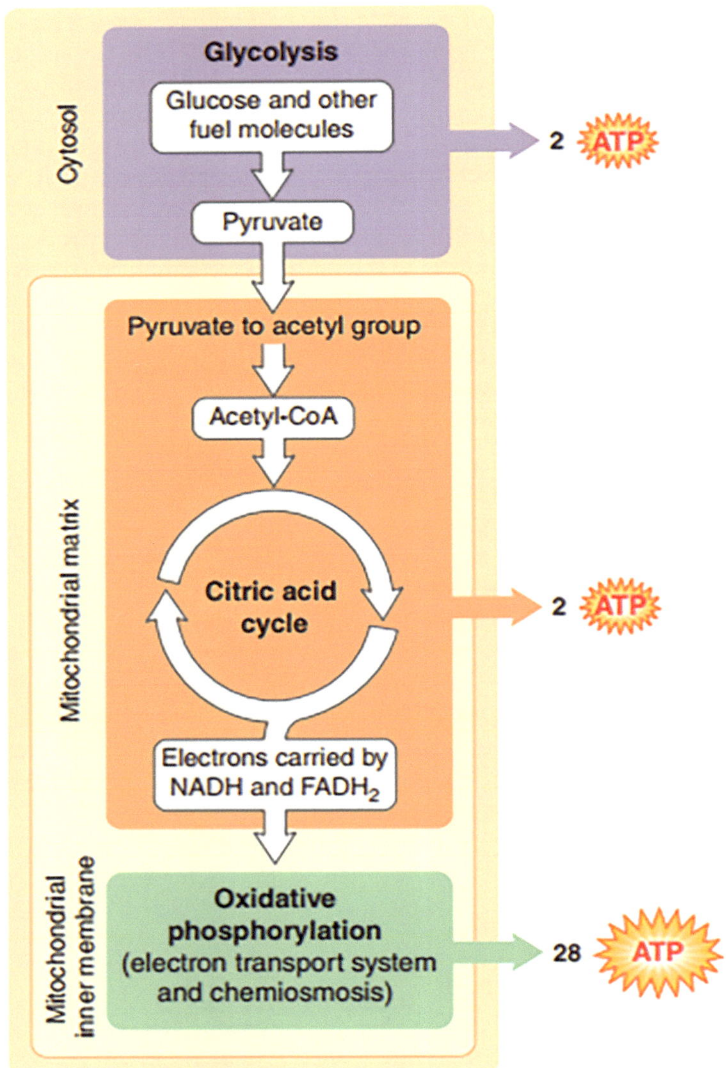

Figure 2.
Energy metabolism [15].

gluconeogenesis. The glycogen reserves in muscle and liver are sufficient to provide 2000 kcal, equivalent to running approximately 32.187 kilometers in a normal person. This amount of energy is generally enough for regular physical exercise, but insufficient for activities like marathon running, where energy is sourced from stored fats [14].

In various studies, after 30 minutes of aerobic physical exercise, the concentration of free fatty acids in the blood significantly increases. This indicates that from the 30-minute mark, fats start to mobilize from adipose tissue. However, the breakdown of fatty acids is slower compared to glucose metabolism through glycolysis. Therefore, the energy formation mechanism in muscles involves a combination of fatty acids and glucose. During low-intensity physical exercise, the largest energy source for ATP production comes from fats, given that more than 30 minutes have passed. In contrast, during moderate- to high-intensity physical exercise, the primary source of energy comes from carbohydrates [14].

Aerobic exercise and endurance training are highly effective in improving physical performance. Aerobic exercise increases fat and glycogen stores in muscle fibers, allowing for a large reserve of energy in the muscles that can be quickly mobilized. Endurance training transforms fast-twitch glycolytic muscle fibers into fast-twitch oxidative-glycolytic fibers [14].

3. Cardiovascular response to physical exercise

At rest, the heart pumps about 5–5.8 L/minute of blood. During heavy activity or physical exercise, cardiac output can drastically increase. In individuals with a sedentary lifestyle, cardiac output during intense activity can reach 20 L/minute. However, trained individuals can experience a 6- to 8-fold increase, reaching 40 L/minute. Oxygen delivery is a crucial factor in determining physical exercise capacity, as seen in scientific studies on exercise metabolism. Those who engage in gradual, sustained, and continuous physical exercise can handle more strenuous workouts than untrained individuals. Heart rate (HR) calculation becomes a crucial variable related to the measurement formula for physical exercise capacity [16].

During physical exercise, the oxygen and nutrient requirements in muscles increase. At rest, skeletal muscles receive about a quarter of the cardiac output, plus 1.2 L/minute. During heavy activity or intense physical exercise, an estimated 88% of the cardiac output is directed to the active muscles. The combination of increased cardiac output and vasodilation in the target muscles allows blood flow to reach 22 L/minute. Vasodilation in active muscles is followed by vasoconstriction in other tissues due to sympathetic signals, but as the muscles become more active, changes occur in the microenvironment of muscle tissue, such as a decrease in tissue O2 concentration and an increase in temperature, CO_2, and interstitial fluid acidity. These factors act as paracrines, causing local vasodilation that can replace sympathetic signals for vasoconstriction [15].

3.1 Ventilatory response to physical exercise

When physical exercise begins and muscles start moving, mechanoreceptors and proprioceptors in the muscles and joints send information about body movement to the motor cortex of the brain. This pathway is excited, and signals travel to the respiratory control center in the medulla oblongata. In response to the movement of physical exercise, the existing signals increase ventilation to maintain oxygen supply as a consequence of increased oxygen utilization [14, 17, 18].

Muscle contractions continue and sensory information provides feedback to the respiratory control that the active body is sufficiently supplied with oxygen and nutrients. Involved sensory receptors include central chemoreceptors, carotid and aortic chemoreceptors, joint proprioceptors, as well as receptors in the muscles, to monitor PO2, PCO2, and pH [18].

Hyperventilation occurring during activity increases proportionally with the intensity of the activity performed. This hyperventilation helps to maintain arterial PO2 and PCO2 close to normal levels. This compensation is crucial and operates effectively, so when monitoring arterial PO2, PCO2, and pH during activity, even heading toward high levels, these parameters do not show significant changes [18].

The K+ ion factor also affects signals. Even during light-intensity activities, extracellular K+ increases with repeated action potentials in muscle fibers, allowing K+ ions to exit the cells. The movement of K+ ions is well captured by carotid chemoreceptors to increase ventilation and balance with the metabolic needs during activity [18].

3.2 Physical activity intensity

The intensity of exercise and physical activity depends significantly on individual factors such as fitness status, age, health status, genetics, psychological factors, social aspects, and exercise habits. Exercise that is too heavy or too light will not contribute to improving an individual's fitness, meaning it will not enhance the ability to consume oxygen per unit time (VO2max). A study suggests that to achieve 95–100% VO2max, an individual needs to engage in regular physical exercise with high intensity. An alternative to the commonly used assessment of VO2max to evaluate an individual's physical activity intensity is heart rate. This is supported by research by Schantz et al. [19] which indicates a close relationship between heart rate and estimating an individual's oxygen consumption. Heart rate and percentage of oxygen consumption capacity are also equivalent in determining the level of an individual's physical activity intensity (**Table 1**).

The commonly used formula to calculate the maximum heart rate is 220 minus age, but this formula may yield values that are either lower or higher than the actual ones. Consequently, several other formulas, which have undergone specific regression in various studies, are available [11]. In cases where individuals have disabilities involving thoracolumbar spinal nerve paralysis and engage in physical activities primarily using their arms, such as propelling a wheelchair, a lower constant of 200 minus age is employed [20].

Intensity	%HRR atau %VO_2R	%HR_{maks}	% VO_2maks
Very low	< 20	< 50	< 37
Low	20–39	50–63	37–45
Moderate	40–59	64–76	46–64
High	60–84	77–93	64–91
Very high	≥ 85	≥ 94	≥ 91
Maximum	100	100	

Table 1.
Physical activity estimation method [19].

Various studies concur on a linear relationship or a direct proportion between heart rate and oxygen consumption capacity in assessing an individual's fitness. These studies were conducted across different levels of physical activity intensity. The correlation remains valid at high intensities; however, at extremely low levels of physical activity intensity, the heart rate may exaggerate an individual's fitness value [21].

4. Concept of maximum oxygen uptake capacity

Fitness measurement is established using the measurement of oxygen consumption per unit time (VO2max). The most common formula is expressed in ($L.kg^{-1}.min^{-1}$). VO2max is the product of maximum cardiac output (CO) or maximal cardiac output ($L.blood.min^{-1}$) and the difference in oxygen levels between the arterial and venous blood ($mLO^2.L.blood^{-1}$). Oxygen consumption is an agreed-upon measure of cellular respiration, expressed in liters of oxygen consumed every minute. The greater the VO2max value, the greater an individual's ability to engage in activities. Up to a certain point, an individual has the ability to continue physical exercise or stop the physical exercise due to fatigue or other factors such as breathlessness, headache, dizziness, or pain. Factors limiting aerobic physical exercise include:

1. The cardiovascular system's ability to supply oxygen and nutrients to tissues,

2. The respiratory system's ability to supply oxygen to the blood, and

3. The muscle's ability to acquire and use oxygen and nutrients efficiently.

Cellular oxygenation occurs within the mitochondria, so the use of oxygen in producing ATP is greatly influenced by the number of mitochondria in the cell. According to physiological studies, muscle metabolism is proven to supply only up to submaximal exercise; in other words, it cannot meet maximal physical exercise activities. Additional energy from outside the muscle and the ability to oxygenate cells are required if someone aims to achieve physical exercise beyond submaximal levels. Increasing the number of mitochondria in muscle cells can be achieved through measured, gradual, continuous, and purposeful exercise that can be accounted for. The transportation of oxygen to each cell in the body heavily depends on the hemoglobin levels in the blood. The normal average hemoglobin level in blood is 15 g/dL for adult males and 14 g/dL for adult females. In addition to hemoglobin levels, it is essential to know the value of oxygen saturation or SaO2. Oxygen saturation indicates the amount of hemoglobin bound to oxygen for transport throughout the body. The normal value of oxygen saturation in average arteries is above 97% [16].

5. Application of cardiorespiratory testing in physical activities

The Duke Activity Status Index is a form commonly used to assess the level of physical activity in terms of metabolic equivalents (METs). A value of 1 MET represents the oxygen consumption of an adult at rest, which is 3.5 $L.kg^{-1}.min^{-1}$ for a person weighing 70 kg in a sitting position. Every active individual should achieve at least a value of 4 METs. An example of daily activities equivalent to this is climbing 12–13 stairs [16].

The use of cardiopulmonary exercise testing (CPET) is non-invasive and low-risk yet remains accurate for assessing heart, lung, and metabolic functions. During this test, the CPET device is utilized throughout the examination while engaging in physical activities. With increasing workload and time, the output of ventilation gas (VE), oxygen consumption (VO2), and carbon dioxide production per minute will increase. Additionally, there will be an observed increase in the accumulation of lactic acid in the muscles [18].

The CPET device can measure the achievement of maximum oxygen consumption per unit time (L/kgBW/min), also known as VO2max. VO2max is the product of maximum cardiac output and the difference in oxygen levels between the arterial and venous blood. VO2max is considered a criterion for measuring physical fitness as it is closely related to the functional capacity of the heart, lungs, and muscles. Some literature also indicates a direct correlation between achieving VO2max and achieving maximum heart rate (HRmax) [11].

The anaerobic threshold (AT) can be considered an estimate of the onset of anaerobic metabolism induced by lactic acidosis levels. This occurs due to an imbalance between the required oxygen supply and the oxygen available in the muscles during activity. While this measurement is rarely invasive, it can be detected on the CPET monitor when the individual exhales an increased amount of CO_2 as compensation for the rise in lactic acidosis levels. The point at which the oxygen consumption curve inverts with the production of VCO2 and VE is the point where lactic acid levels rapidly increase. This point is captured by CPET as the VO2max value for that individual. VO2max also correlates with gender, age, body weight, and the intensity of a specific activity [22].

CPET: research conducted by the author using CPET equipment in 2015 showed that the highest VO2max value in a group of post injured soldiers (PIS) propelling wheelchairs was 38 L/min/kgBW, while for normal soldier (NS) engaged in running, it was 64 L/min/kgBW. In other words, the VO2max value in the group of PIS propelling wheelchairs only reached 45% compared to soldiers running [20]. By investigating the equivalence of VO2max between running and wheelchair-propelling activities for soldiers post-injury who cannot or eventually cannot run again, an equivalence value can be sought to assess physical ability.

6. Effects of immobilization and inactive musculoskeletal system

The state of immobilization or a sedentary lifestyle will lead to a loss of strength, commonly known as a decrease in muscle strength, which ultimately reduces the strength and tolerance of physical endurance for daily activities. During total bed rest for a duration of 1 week, muscle strength and endurance tolerance will decrease by 10–15% from the initial strength. Even in healthy individuals undergoing bed rest for more than 5 weeks, losses can persist, reaching up to 35–50%. Research involving dynamic leg press during the immobilization period showed that extensor and flexor strength of the knee could be maintained, but the strength of the plantar flexors of the ankle and dorsiflexors of the ankle could not be sustained. Therefore, the best exercises are functional walking or mobilization. In conclusion, muscle atrophy resulting from disuse is more evident in the legs than in the arms. Studies on individuals with total bed rest indicate a strength decrease of 20–40% in the legs, while a decrease of only +5% occurs in the arms. The decrease in myofibril strength per unit volume of muscle fibers appears to be reduced [12].

The loss of strength and muscle mass will continue to decline until the individual finds it difficult to rise from an immobilized state. Exercises can be done gradually, continuously, and sustainably, with quantifiable and justifiable progress. To reverse the effects of immobilization syndrome after 45 days, functional mobilization exercises and electrical stimulation therapy assistance for around 45 days can be employed to maintain the ability to return to basic mobility [12].

Immobilization syndrome has also been proven to decrease muscle endurance due to a decrease in the concentration of ATP and muscle glycogen reserves. Decreases in muscle protein synthesis, oxidative enzyme function, acceleration into the anaerobic cycle, and the accumulation of lactic acid are a set of factors leading to the onset of fatigue. Changes in the shape and size of motor end-plates and dysfunction of acetylcholine receptors further impair the function of skeletal muscle endurance. The reduced oxygen demand of muscles during immobilization significantly affects the number and size of mitochondria.

After 42 days of immobilization, there is a 16% reduction in VO2max, a decrease in cardiac output by up to 30%, a 40% reduction in oxygen transport flow, and a 28% reduction in mitochondrial volume [12].

6.1 High intensity interval training (HIIT)

Since the 1950s, Olympic athletes have been introduced to HIIT as one of the exercises to enhance their performance. The first introduced interval training was sprint interval training, where athletes perform exercises reaching 100% of their maximal heart rate (HR), followed by a gradual descent. This cycle is repeated several times. According to a survey conducted by the American College of Sports Medicine in 2014, HIIT has become popular among the general public. This exercise takes 30 minutes, including both aerobic and resistance training phases with vigorous intensity [20, 23, 24].

Research using mice aims to prove whether high-intensity interval training (HIIT) and/or moderate-intensity continuous training (MICT) can contribute to or even enhance cardioprotection. In the mechanism of increasing Klotho protein and reducing TRPC6 (which, when increased, causes stress and leads to dysfunction and heart diseases), some studies show that the cardioprotective factor in patients with myocardial ischemia-reperfusion (IR) is highly influenced by the intensity of exercise rather than the duration of exercise [20, 23–26].

HIIT is an exercise with a repetitive pattern at high intensity, reaching 85–90% peak VO2. HIIT starts with a 5-minute warm-up achieving 40–50% of the maximum heart rate (low intensity). Entering the core of the HIIT exercise for 6 × 2 minutes (with high intensity at 85–90% of the maximum heart rate) is interspersed with 5 × 2 minutes (with low intensity at 50–60% of the maximum heart rate), known as the active recovery period. It concludes with a 5-minute cooling down period with an intensity of 40–50% of the maximum heart rate. On the other hand, MICT begins with a 5-minute warm-up at 40–50% of the maximum heart rate and concludes with a 5-minute cooling down period at a low intensity. The core exercise reaches 70% of the maximum heart rate. MICT exercises should be performed for a minimum of 30 minutes [27–29].

This study successfully noted that after all experimental animals performed exercises for five consecutive days, there was a reduction in the size of the infarct area compared to mice without physical exercise. Moreover, it turns out that HIIT exercises have a more positive effect compared to MICT. Thus, it can be concluded that, despite short-term aerobic exercise training in IR patients, it has a positive effect as a trigger for cardioprotection [30–32].

6.2 The relationship between exercise and immune system

Research on the connection between physical performance and the immune system has significantly evolved since the 1900s and continues to progress [33]. The current focus remains on three aspects:

1. Reducing fat, especially visceral fat.

2. Increasing the production of the immune system's building blocks. Lowering the risk of diseases such as diabetes, heart disease, and stroke by up to 80% [34].

3. Releasing anti-inflammatory or anti-cytokine substances resulting from the contraction of skeletal muscles [35].

6.3 Measured exercise

To determine the intensity of the exercise we engage in, we need to calculate our age, measure our pulse, and refer to a table estimating physical activity. For example:

Age: 50 years, then use the formula: 200–50 (age) = 170 (Maximum heart rate).

(A)

Check your pulse while exercising, count for 1 minute. Suppose it's 150 beats/minute.

(B)

Calculate the intensity: (achieved pulse (B) 150) / (maximum pulse (A) 170) = 88% intensity.

Check the **Table 2**.

After referring to the table above, it turns out that it falls into the heavy intensity category [33, 36].

Frequency: The recommended frequency for physical activity is 5 days a week.

This is an ideal frequency. To ensure that your exercise provides optimal immune system benefits, it is recommended to exercise at least three times a week, with an optimal frequency of five times a week, allowing the body to experience rest for energy restoration [33, 36].

Time: the recommended daily exercise duration is a minimum of 30 minutes to 60 minutes. Based on the breakdown of fat after moderate-intensity exercise for

Intensity	% Maximum heart rate
Very light	< 57
Light	57 – <64
Moderate	64 – <76
Hard	76 – <96
Very hard	≥ 96

Table 2.
Estimation table of daily activity.

Monday	Tuesday	Wednesday	Thursday	Friday	Saturday	Sunday
Light intensity + muscle strengthening	Moderate intensity	Rest day	Moderate intensity	Light intensity + muscle strengthening	Heavy intensity	Rest day
Brisk walk + weight lifting for 60 minutes	Light jogging for 60 minutes		Light jogging for 60 minutes	Light dancing + weight lifting for 45 minutes	Running/ cycling/ swimming/ golf	

Table 3.
Types of exercises.

30 minutes, exercising for 4 hours a week reduces the risk of diabetes, stroke, and heart attacks by 80% [33, 34, 36].

Type: various types of exercises can be chosen.

a. Aerobic: exercises that consistently use oxygen in every movement, characterized by not getting too breathless. Examples include walking, jogging, dancing, cycling, swimming, and golf.

b. Anaerobic: high speed, short-duration exercises, such as sprinting 100 m or chasing a ball in soccer with high speed for a short time, repeated.

c. Muscle strengthening: using weights or body weight as resistance [33, 36].

After understanding FITT (frequency, intensity, time, and type), you can combine them. If you find it challenging to maintain heavy intensity for 5 days a week, especially at a very high level, you can combine FITT elements according to your capability. See **Table 3**, for example.

7. Conclusion

1. Moderate to heavy-intensity exercise with the right FITT will enhance immunity to improve health status, physical fitness, and quality of life.

2. Very low or very high-intensity exercises with very long durations can be detrimental to health status, physical fitness, and quality of life [34, 36].

3. Always consider your overall health condition, age, monitor your heart rate during exercise, time, and the type of exercise you engage in.

4. This exercise prescription is unique to each individual. Consult with a doctor if you have any underlying health conditions.

Here is an example of a study to establish a home program with important limitations that are easily understood by the community.

How likely is it for a post-leg injury patient to exercise with a wheelchair? Can wheelchair exercise be turned into a home program? These questions often arise in the minds of physiotherapists when encountering individuals with leg injuries who still require assistive devices for ambulation. The following facts from a wheelchair sports exercise test conducted on normal soldiers (NS) and injured and post-injured soldier (PIS) will be presented. This can help physiotherapists make decisions and establish criteria that can be implemented for injured patients still in need of ambulatory aids, using a wheelchair as a means of exercise to maintain the fitness of patients or individuals with disabilities [37].

Serving in the military comes with the risk of injuries, and data from the Rehabilitation Center (Pusrehab) from 2009 to December 2018 recorded 6640 post-injured soldiers. This accounts for approximately 1.66% of all active soldiers to date [37]. About 75% of them suffered injuries from the lumbar region downward. This significantly affects the physical condition of soldiers returning to duty, especially in combat or sports, depending on their functional abilities. To fulfill the country's obligation to protect its citizens, especially injured and post injured military personnel (PIS), the Rehabilitation Center of the Ministry of Defense of the Republic of Indonesia (PUSREHAB) was established to provide comprehensive medical rehabilitation services [38].

In the second semester of 2021, PUSREHAB conducted medical rehabilitation for 75 male PIS, with an average injury duration of 4 years. A total of 50 of them have undergone evaluation using a wheelchair exercise test. At the same time, 104 male NS also underwent the wheelchair exercise test. All evaluations were approved by Pusrehab and Pusdikkes KodiklatAD. A total of 154 active, healthy male soldiers who had undergone a prior Medical Check-Up (MCU) stating no acute infectious diseases or uncontrolled illnesses were selected. Subjects with balanced arm capabilities for wheelchair exercise were chosen for this test, using a sports wheelchair (**Figures 3** and **4**) [38].

Looking at the results of **Table 4** to assess the general characteristics, no significant differences were found between PIS and NS. When the data are grouped per 10 years of age, there are significant differences for the age group of 19 to 29 years in terms of age, body weight, and BMI. The PIS age for this group is senior compared to NS. The BMI reaches 28 (obesity category 1) [38]. This almost homogeneous data will simplify data analysis.

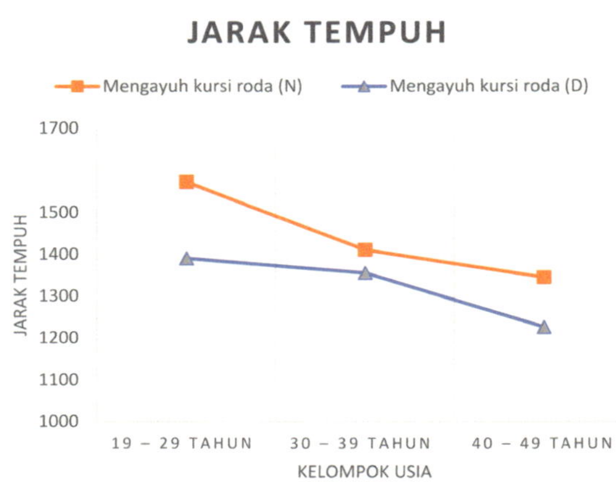

Figure 3.
Distance traveled using wheelchair.

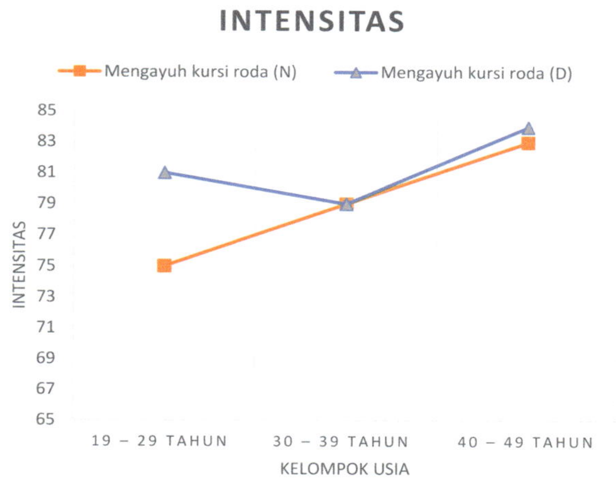

Figure 4.
Exercise intensity using wheelchair.

From the conducted tests, differences were found in the results of this fitness evaluation. As seen in **Table 4**, there are significant differences in the distance covered in the wheelchair exercise test between PIS and NS. In general, there is a mean difference of 117 meters, with NS covering a greater distance than PIS. When classified into age groups, the differences in distance are: for 19–29 years, 182 meters; for 30–39 years, 55 meters; and for the age group of 40–49 years, 118 meters. The results show that, in all age groups, NS covers a greater distance than PIS. It is clear that as age increases, the covered distance decreases. This happens in both groups. The difference in covered distance between NS and PIS indicates different fitness results for these two groups. NS appears to be superior to PIS.

Qi and colleagues state that the functional speed wheelchair distance is 720–936 meters per 12 minutes [39]. When compared with the achievements in this evaluation for the age groups of 19–29, 30–39, and 40–49 years (1555, 1400, 1330 m), it can be said that they have entered the exercise range.

An interesting aspect is the intensity of the exercise achieved during the data collection. All subjects performed this test with moderate intensity in the age group under 40. However, those above 40 years, entered vigorous intensity, but none of the subjects reached maximal intensity. Observations of the intensity of wheelchair exercise performed by soldiers under 40 can still be considered safe since it is within the moderate range. For those above 40, it is also considered safe but should be done with caution because it reaches an average intensity of 83% (heavy intensity). Therefore, recording the pulse during the activity can be used as one of the benchmarks for a home program exercise independently [39].

From the two data sets above, it can be seen that as a person ages, more effort is needed to perform activities, as shown by the increased intensity of activities, although the covered distance will decrease. In other words, a person's fitness will decline with age. This aligns with the aging journal, which states a decrease in VO2peak by 3–6% per decade starting at the age of 30–40 years [40].

In conclusion, the fitness outcomes for post-injured soldiers (PIS) continue to lag behind those of Normal Soldiers (NS), underscoring the necessity for comprehensive medical rehabilitation programs for every post-injured soldier. The distance covered and pulse rate attained during wheelchair exercise serve as reliable indicators for

Variable	Age	Normal soldier $n = 104$	Post injured soldier $n = 50$	Sig.
Age (years)		32 (19–49)	31 (23–51)	0.404
	19–29	22 (19–29)	26 ± 2	0.000*
	30–39	33 (31–38)	35 ± 3	0.072
	40–49	44 ± 3	44. ± 4	0.721
Weight (kg)		69.7 ± 8.2	72.18 ± 10.55	0.241
	19–29	64.1 ± 8	69.8 ± 10.7	0.016*
	30–39	75.1 ± 5.8	75.1 ± 11.2	0.994
	40–49	72.1 ± 4.9	72.4 ± 8	0.884
Height (cm)		170 (163–183)	169.6 ± 4.0	0.866
	19–29	169.1 ± 4.1	170 ± 3.9	0.432
	30–39	170.7 ± 4.6	169.7 ± 4.7	0.302
	40–49	168.5 ± 3.9	168.4 ± 3	0.922
Body mass index (BMI) (Kg/m^2)		24.22 ± 2.5	24.67 ± 5.0	0.393
	19–29	22.3 ± 2.2	24.2 ± 3.8	0.044*
	30–39	26.3 (20–29)	25.8 ± 1.7	0.893
	40–49	25.6 (21–27)	25.5 ± 2.5	0.847
Blood pressure (systole) (mmHg)		120 (90–146)	123.86 ± 13.5	0.455
	19–29	120 ± 12	121 ± 10	0.989
	30–39	120 (98–130)	123 ± 13	0.275
	40–49	125 ± 12	133 ± 19	0.151
Blood pressure (diastole) (mmHg)		80 (58–100)	78.92 ± 7.4	0.617
	19–29	73 (58–100)	77 ± 7	0.088
	30–39	81 ± 8	80 ± 7	0.791
	40–49	80 (67–91)	82 ± 9	0.937
Hemoglobin (g/dL)		15.0 ± 1.3	14.9 ± 1.1	0.550
	19–29	14.8 ± 1.2	15 ± 1	0.644
	30–39	15.3 ± 1.3	14.9 ± 1.3	0.324
	40–49	15 ± 1.4	14.7 ± 1.1	0.536
Blood sugar (g/dL)		95.8 ± 15.9	92.5 (74 ± 391)	0.914
	19–29	95 ± 18	88 (77–121)	0.488
	30–39	95 ± 15	96 (70–126)	0465
	40–49	98 ± 15	101 (89–391)	0.395

Table 4.
Subject characteristic.

assessing the safety of patients engaging in such activities. Moreover, the pulse rates achieved during these exercises fall within the moderate category, indicating that they remain safe for individuals recovering from injuries. These findings emphasize the importance of tailored rehabilitation efforts and ongoing monitoring to ensure the well-being and progress of post-injury patients, particularly those utilizing wheelchairs as part of their exercise regimen.

Exercise is Medicine
DOI: http://dx.doi.org/10.5772/intechopen.1005262

Author details

Endang Ernandini* and Jonathan Alvin Wiryaputra
Medical Faculty of Republic Indonesia, Defense University, Indonesia

*Address all correspondence to: ernandiniebeb@gmail.com

References

[1] Dapp LC, Gashaj V, Roebers CM. Physical activity and motor skills in children: A differentiated approach. Psychology of Sport and Exercise. 2021;**54**:101916

[2] Robinson LE, Stodden DF, Barnett LM, Lopes VP, Logan SW, Rodrigues LP, et al. Motor competence and its effect on positive developmental trajectories of health. Sports Medicine. 2015;**45**:1273-1284

[3] Hebert JJ, Klakk H, Møller NC, Grøntved A, Andersen LB, Wedderkopp N. The prospective association of organized sports participation with cardiovascular disease risk in children (the CHAMPS study-DK). Mayo Clinic Proceedings. 2017;**92**(1):57-65

[4] Ruiz JR, Ortega FB, Castillo R, Martín-Matillas M, Kwak L, Vicente-Rodríguez G, et al. Physical activity, fitness, weight status, and cognitive performance in adolescents. The Journal of Pediatrics. 2010;**157**(6):917-922

[5] Barkley RA, Knouse LE, Murphy KR. Correspondence and disparity in the self-and other ratings of current and childhood ADHD symptoms and impairment in adults with ADHD. Psychological Assessment. 2011;**23**(2):437

[6] Thompson WR, Sallis R, Joy E, Jaworski CA, Stuhr RM, Trilk JL. Exercise is medicine. American Journal of Lifestyle Medicine. 2020;**14**(5):511-523

[7] Heissel A, Heinen D, Brokmeier LL, Skarabis N, Kangas M, Vancampfort D, et al. Exercise as medicine for depressive symptoms? A systematic review and meta-analysis with meta-regression. British Journal of Sports Medicine. 2023;**57**(16):1049-1057

[8] Izquierdo M, Merchant RA, Morley JE, Anker SD, Aprahamian I, Arai H, et al. International exercise recommendations in older adults (ICFSR): Expert consensus guidelines. The Journal of Nutrition, Health & Aging. 2021;**25**(7):824-853

[9] D'Onofrio G, Kirschner J, Prather H, Goldman D, Rozanski A. Musculoskeletal exercise: Its role in promoting health and longevity. Progress in Cardiovascular Diseases. 2023;**77**:25-36

[10] Thyfault JP, Bergouignan A. Exercise and metabolic health: Beyond skeletal muscle. Diabetologia. 2020;**63**(8):1464-1474

[11] Cohen J. A power primer. Psychological Bulletin. 1992;**112**(1): 155-159

[12] Ernandini E, Pakasi TA. Physical fitness profile of wheelchair-bound soldier: A preliminary study to propose a new standard for disabled soldier. Indonesian Journal of Physical Medicine and Rehabilitation. 2020;**9**(2):11-18

[13] Gil-Garcia JR. Using partial least squares in digital government research. In: Garson GD, Khosrow-Pour DBAM, editors. Handbook of Research on Public Information Technology [Internet]. IGI Global; 2008. pp. 239-253. Available from: http://services.igi-global.com/resolvedoi/resolve.aspx?doi=10.4018/978-1-59904-857-4.ch023 [Accessed: Jul 5, 2022]

[14] Sherwood L. Human Physiology: From Cells to Systems. 7th ed. Belmont, CA: Brooks/Cole, Cengage Learning; 2010

[15] Henseler J, Ringle C, Sarstedt M. A new criterion for assessing discriminant validity in variance-based structural equation Modeling. Journal of the Academy of Marketing Science. 2015;**43**:115-135

[16] Liguzinski P, Korzeniewski B. Oxygen delivery by blood determines the maximal VO2 and work rate during whole body exercise in humans: in silico studies. American Journal of Physiology. Heart and Circulatory Physiology. 2007;**293**(1):H343-H353

[17] Le van den A, Holla JFM, Dadema T, Visser B, Valent LJ, de Groot S, et al. Determinants of physical activity in wheelchair users with spinal cord injury or lower limb amputation: Perspectives of rehabilitation professionals and wheelchair users. Disability and Rehabilitation [Internet]. 2020;**42**(14). Available from: https://pubmed.ncbi.nlm.nih.gov/30924706/

[18] Boone T. Introduction to Exercise Physiology. Jones & Bartlett Publishers; 2014. 577 p

[19] Tran D. Cardiopulmonary exercise testing. In: Guest PC, editor. Investigations of Early Nutrition Effects on Long-Term Health [Internet], Methods in Molecular Biology. Vol. 1735. Available from: http://link.springer.com/10.1007/978-1-4939-7614-0_18. New York, NY: Springer New York; 2018. pp. 285-295 [Accessed: Jul 1, 2022]

[20] Powers SK, Smuder AJ, Kavazis AN, Quindry JC. Mechanisms of exercise-induced cardioprotection. Physiology. 2014;**29**(1):27-38

[21] Presiden Republik Indonesia, Dewan Perwakilan Rakyat Indonesia. Undang-Undang Nomor 34 Tahun 2004 tentang Tentara Nasional Indonesia. 2004. 0-42 p

[22] Ghozali I. Structural Equation Modeling Metode Alternatif Dengan Partial Least Squares (PLS). 4th ed. Semarang: Universitas Diponegoro; 2014

[23] Quindry J, Hamilton KL. Exercise and cardiac preconditioning against ischemia reperfusion injury. Current Cardiology Reviews. 2013;**9**(3):220-229

[24] Ikeda G, Matoba T, Nakano Y, Nagaoka K, Ishikita A, Nakano K, et al. Nanoparticle-mediated targeting of cyclosporine a enhances cardioprotection against ischemia-reperfusion injury through inhibition of mitochondrial permeability transition pore opening. Scientific Reports. 2016;**6**:20467

[25] Borges JP, Lessa MA. Mechanisms involved in exercise-induced cardioprotection: A systematic review. Arquivos Brasileiros de Cardiologia. 2015;**105**(1):71-81

[26] Morciano G, Preti D, Pedriali G, Aquila G, Missiroli S, Fantinati A, et al. Discovery of novel 1, 3, 8-triazaspiro [4.5] decane derivatives that target the c subunit of F1/FO-adenosine triphosphate (ATP) synthase for the treatment of reperfusion damage in myocardial infarction. Journal of Medicinal Chemistry. 2018;**61**(16):7131-7143

[27] Xie J, Cha S-K, An S-W, Kuro-o M, Birnbaumer L, Huang C-L. Cardioprotection by klotho through downregulation of TRPC6 channels in the mouse heart. Nature Communications. 2012;**3**:1238

[28] Mencke R, Olauson H, Hillebrands J-L. Effects of klotho on fibrosis and cancer: A renal focus on mechanisms and therapeutic strategies. Advanced Drug Delivery Reviews. 2017;**121**:85-100

[29] Guiraud T, Nigam A, Gremeaux V, Meyer P, Juneau M, Bosquet L.

High-intensity interval training in cardiac rehabilitation. Sports Medicine. 2012;**42**(7):587-605

[30] Rognmo Ø, Moholdt T, Bakken H, Hole T, Mølstad P, Myhr NE, et al. Cardiovascular risk of high-versus moderate-intensity aerobic exercise in coronary heart disease patients. Circulation. 2012;**112**:123117

[31] Swain DP, Franklin BA. Comparison of cardioprotective benefits of vigorous versus moderate intensity aerobic exercise. The American Journal of Cardiology. 2006;**97**:141-147

[32] Rankin A, Rankin A, MacIntyre P, Hillis W. Walk or run? Is high-intensity exercise more effective than moderate-intensity exercise at reducing cardiovascular risk? Scottish Medical Journal. 2012;**57**:99-102

[33] R. Frontera W. DeLisa's Physical Medicine & Rehabilitation: Principles and Practice. 5th ed. Philadelphia: Lippincott Williams & Wilkins; 2010

[34] Gleeson M et al. The Anti-Inflammatory Effects of Exercise: Mechanisms and Implications for the Prevention and Treatment of Disease. Loughborough University, UK. Published online 5 August 2011

[35] Sherwood L. Human Physiology: From Cells to Systems. 9th ed. Vol. 3. Boston; 2016

[36] Riebe D. In: Riebe D, editor. ACSM's Guidelines for Exercise Testing and Prescription. 10th ed. Wolters Kluwer; 2018

[37] Pertahanan K. Keputusan Menteri Pertahanan No. Kep/365/M/IX/2019 tentang Penyelenggaraan Rehabilitasi Terpadu bagi Penyandang Disabilitas Personel TNI dan PNS Kemhan dan Rehabilitasi Medik Paripurna Return to Combat bagi Penyandang Disabilitas Personel TNI. 2019

[38] Litbangkes Kementerian Kesehatan. Hasil Utama RISKESDAS. 2018

[39] Qi L, Ferguson-Pell M, Salimi Z, Haennel R, Ramadi A. Wheelchair users' perceived exertion during typical mobility activities. Spinal Cord. 2015;**53**(9):687-691

[40] Jackson AS, Sui X, Hébert JR, Church TS, Blair SN. Role of lifestyle and aging on the longitudinal change in cardiorespiratory fitness. Archives of Internal Medicine. 2009;**169**(19):1781-1787

Section 2

Exercise Medicine for Specific Health Conditions

Chapter 4

Effect and Improvement of Lifestyle Intervention on Hyperlipidemia

Shan Gao and Zuowei Pei

Abstract

The study found that the abdominal circumference, body mass index, blood pressure, and blood lipid levels of the patients were significantly decreased after the healthy lifestyle intervention, and the proportion of smoking and alcohol abuse was significantly reduced. Healthy lifestyle intervention has become the key content of guiding the treatment of hyperlipidemia. Therefore, this chapter will briefly introduce the main pathogenic factors of hyperlipidemia in daily life, and then introduce the impact factors and improvement effect of lifestyle intervention on hyperlipidemia from four aspects of diet, exercise, psychological factors and risk factors in detail.

Keywords: hyperlipidemia, dietary, exercise, psychology, lifestyle, prevention

1. Introduction

With the advancement of people's living conditions and technology, more and more sub-healthy phenomena have emerged in people's body, which leads to many diseases. Among them, hyperlipidemia means an imbalance between the levels of low-density lipoprotein cholesterol (LDL-C) and high-density lipoprotein cholesterol (HDL-C) in the blood, including hypertriglyceridemia and mixed hyperlipidemia, in which both total cholesterol (TC) and total triglyceride (TG) levels are elevated [1]. As one of the most commonly found and treated diseases in dyslipidemia, hyperlipidemia will be associated with cardiovascular diseases such as atherosclerosis [2]. Studies show that cardiovascular disease (CVD) is one of the leading causes of death among adults in the U.S. Compared to people with normal TC levels, people with hyperlipidemia have about twice the risk of developing CVD [3]. It poses a great risk to people's health. Current clinical results show that few patients need drugs to lower TG and TC levels, and that lifestyle changes are the most effective way to improve hyperlipidemia [4].

Daily life interventions can improve hyperlipidemia in several ways: diet, exercise, psychological factors, and elimination of risk factors. Studies have shown that chronic high-calorie diets exhibit hyperinsulinemia and hyperlipidemia, as well as heavier body and gonadal fat weights [5]. Conversely, moderate rise in aerobic exercise and physical activity elevate HDL-C levels while reducing LDL-C, TC, and TG, thereby exerting a positive impact on patients with hyperlipidemia [6]. When there is a mood disorder, cholesterol levels may be affected by the acute mood state and thus change. There is evidence that cholesterol levels are elevated when depressive episodes occur, suggesting that the effect of mood states on cholesterol levels does also exist [7]. In addition, some poor lifestyles and habits as well as common diseases can also increase the risk of dyslipidemia. Over the past few decades, there has been a notable rise in the incidence of cardiometabolic risk (CMR) factors, including central obesity, insulin resistance, hypertension, and dyslipidemia, among individuals with type 1 diabetes. These factors may have an additive or synergistic effect on the risk of developing cardiovascular disease. This suggests that individuals with type 1 diabetes should not only focus on managing their blood sugar levels but also take measures to control other CMR factors to minimize their overall cardiovascular risk. Specifically, for individuals with multiple CMR factors, more aggressive interventions such as regular physical exercise, healthy dietary habits, and pharmacotherapy may be necessary [8].

Therefore, daily life interventions may have a positive impact on lipid levels in patients with hyperlipidemia and may be more effective as adjunctive therapy.

2. The effect and improvement of dietary patterns on hyperlipidemia

2.1 Pathological mechanism of hyperlipidemia caused by improper diet

During human metabolism, lipid metabolism is mainly regulated by nutrients such as sugars and fatty acids. Glucose is an essential energy material for normal metabolic activities, while glucose and fructose are the main utilization sugars. Compared with the use of glucose, the consumption of fructose by the body leads to an increase in the level of circulating apolipoprotein C3(Apo C3), which may be due to the failure of fructose to induce insulin secretion, stimulating the expression of Apo C3 and reducing the reverse transport of cholesterol. On the other hand, consumption of a high-glucose diet can induce the expression of Apo C3, which can increase the low-density lipoprotein (LDL) and subsequently impact the hydrolysis of triglycerides (TG) in chylomicrons (CM) and very low-density lipoprotein (VLDL) [9]. Therefore, a high-glucose diet, especially a diet with high fructose content, is a major cause of hyperlipidemia. Specifically, if the proportion of sugar intake is too high, it will increase insulin secretion, resulting in hyperinsulinemia, which promotes the synthesis of triglycerides in the liver, leading to an increase in the concentration of triglycerides in the plasma. In addition, the change in external factors such as high-glucose diet can also induce the increase in Apo C3 gene expression, resulting in the increase in plasma Apo C3 concentration, which will reduce lipoprotein lipase (LPL) activity, and further hinder the hydrolysis of triglycerides in CM and VLDL [9], thus causing hypertriglyceridemia. In general, a diet high in glucose can lead to an increase in blood triglyceride levels, which is a risk factor for hypertriglyceridemia and hyperlipidemia. High levels of blood lipids can increase the risk of developing cardiovascular diseases such as atherosclerosis and heart disease. Therefore, maintaining a reasonable dietary structure, limiting the intake of excess calories, and reducing a high-glucose diet are of great significance for the prevention and treatment of abnormal lipid metabolism.

Fatty acids (FA) are essential nutrients for vital activities and can be divided into saturated fatty acids (SFA) and unsaturated fatty acids (USFA). Animal fats are generally rich in SFA, while trans fatty acids (TFA) are present in butter, whole milk products, and ruminant meat and they are "partially hydrogenated fatty acids" of industrial origin [10]. SFA was the dietary factor that had the greatest effect on LDL-C levels, and LDL-C increased by 0.02–0.04 mmol/L for each 1% increase in energy from saturated fat. Dietary TFA increased LDL-C in a similar manner to SFA, but TFA reduced HDL-C [11]. In addition to the effects on cholesterol levels, lipid metabolism may also be affected by the interaction of dietary lipids with intestinal microflora. This interaction may lead to abnormalities such as lipid metabolism disorders in the body [12]. Hypercholesterolemia is also a common symptom of hyperlipidemia. The synthesis of cholesterol in the body will be promoted due to a diet high in calories, cholesterol, and saturated fatty acids, leading to an increase in liver cholesterol content. In addition, the receptor synthesis of LDL is decreased, and the receptor activity of LDL on the cell surface is further decreased, so that the affinity of LDL with its receptor is decreased, and the cholesterol level in blood is increased. Conversely, if you eat a low-calorie diet, unsaturated fatty acids can affect the activity of enzymes involved in cholesterol synthesis, resulting in lower blood cholesterol levels. Therefore, the FA composition in the diet has an important effect on lipid metabolism and cholesterol level in the body. In daily diet, the intake of USFA should be moderate, and the intake of SFA and TFA should be limited to maintain good lipid metabolism and healthy cholesterol levels.

2.2 Clinical manifestations of hyperlipidemia caused by improper diet

The clinical manifestations of hyperlipidemia caused by improper diet will vary according to the severity of the disease and the types of elevated blood lipids, while hyperlipidemia often causes lesion damage to the heart, brain, skin, and other places. The clinical manifestations are mainly xanthoma, early-onset corneal ring, fundus changes and arteriosclerosis, etc. However, in the majority of early onset, patients have no obvious symptoms and signs [13]. Specifically, common clinical manifestations include the following:

(1) Xanthoma: Xanthoma varies in size and there are small masses as well as large plaques. It occurs frequently in the eyelids, and may occur in the hands, feet, and certain joints. Xanthomas are usually painless, but may cause itching or irritation. Xanthoma is caused by the accumulation of cholesterol in the skin and may be a marker of high LDL-C levels. (2) Rings for the elderly: Rings for the elderly are more common in the elderly and are usually bilateral. It is caused by the deposition of cholesterol in the eye and may be a sign of high cholesterol levels in the blood. The ring around the cornea of the eye is either intact or incomplete. It is more obvious in the upper part of the cornea. Although the ring in the elderly is usually asymptomatic, it may be a sign of potential cardiovascular disease. (3) Retinal hyperlipidemia: It is a rare disease, usually caused by extremely high levels of triglycerides (higher than 1000 mg/dL), which can lead to visual impairment or even blindness if not treated immediately. (4) Peripheral artery disease: High cholesterol levels lead to the accumulation of plaques in the arteries that supply blood to the legs and arms, leading to peripheral artery disease that manifests as leg pain, numbness, and weakness. (5) Abdominal pain: High level of triglyceride will lead to acute pancreatitis, causing severe abdominal pain, nausea, vomiting, and fever. (6) Fatigue: High levels of lipids in the blood lead to fatigue and weakness, but this symptom may be a non-specific symptom of hyperlipidemia. (7) Cardiovascular disease: High levels of LDL-C can lead to the development of atherosclerosis, which can cause CVD, including heart attack and stroke. (8) Hypertension: High level of lipids in blood will lead to hypertension, which is a common complication of hyperlipidemia.

In general, the clinical manifestations of hyperlipidemia caused by poor diet include benign skin diseases to life-threatening CVD. Therefore, timely dietary intervention and regular detection of blood lipid levels are the key to the prevention and treatment of hyperlipidemia and its complications.

2.3 How to change the diet will improve hyperlipidemia

With the deepening of research on hyperlipidemia, in addition to drug treatment, treatment options to improve hyperlipidemia by changing dietary patterns have received more and more attention. These strategies include reducing the intake of cholesterol and saturated fatty acids, and consuming lipid-lowering foods [14, 15]. In daily diet, we should pay attention to control the intake of cholesterol and saturated fatty acids, and eat more foods rich in USFA and reducing blood lipid in order to maintain a good blood lipid level.

1. Eating food rich in dietary fiber (DF) [16] is an effective method for reducing blood lipid. DF refers to the sum of edible plant components, carbohydrates, and similar substances that are resistant to digestion and absorption in the small intestine of the human body but can be partially or completely fermented in the large intestine. According to whether it is soluble in water, it can be divided into soluble cellulose and insoluble cellulose [17]. Studies have shown that common cardiovascular diseases such as hyperlipidemia, hypertension, and coronary heart disease are related to the insufficient intake of DF [18]. DF can increase the fullness of the stomach on the one hand, reduce the intake of energy such as food, and play a role in the prevention of obesity. On the other hand, it can increase gastrointestinal peristalsis, improve the environment of the digestive tract probiotics, and then promote the excretion of toxins in the body, reducing the incidence of high cholesterol [19]. At the same time, DF can play an inhibitory role in the absorption of cholesterol and triglyceride by the lymphatic system, thereby promoting the normal operation of lipid and lipoprotein metabolism in the body. Three plants rich in natural DF, such as radish, beet, and Chinese cabbage, could significantly reduce the triglyceride content in serum and liver and improve the abnormal phenomenon of lipid metabolism in the body [20]. In addition, research has also focused on composite dietary fiber (DFC). The results showed that DFC prepared with sea buckthorn peel, bean gum, and oat bran as the main raw materials had a significant efficacy in reducing blood lipid. In conclusion, intake of food rich in dietary fiber is a natural, mild, and effective method for reducing blood lipid. In daily diet, it is recommended to eat more foods rich in dietary fiber, such as vegetables, fruits, whole grains, in order to maintain a good blood lipid level.

2. The intake of USFA is also an effective method for reducing blood lipid [21]. Compared with the saturated fatty acids in most animal fats and oils, many vegetable oils are rich in a variety of unsaturated fatty acids and have received widespread attention. For example, studies have shown that celery seed oil is rich in unsaturated fatty acids such as palmitic acid, oleic acid, and linoleic acid. On the one hand, it can significantly reduce the levels of TC, TG, and LDL-C in serum of hyperlipidemia and the arteriosclerosis index LDL-C/HDL-C. On the other hand, the activity of superoxide dismutase (SOD) in serum and liver is remarkably improved. It was further proved that celery seed oil could enhance

the activity of antioxidant enzymes, effectively improve the antioxidant level in the body, remove excess free radicals in the body, and avoid the damage of lipid peroxidation and its intermediate metabolites to the body, thereby improving blood lipid metabolism. The camellia seed oil in the vegetable oil can not only reduce the serum TG and TC levels, but also alleviate the fatty lesions in the liver. All of the above are unsaturated fatty acids rich in oil plants; however, the unsaturated fatty acids rich in natural algae cannot be ignored. Studies show that *Chlorella* also has a significant effect on reducing blood lipid and is an option to alleviate hyperlipidemia [21]. In addition to vegetable oils, marine animal fats and oils such as fish also contain unsaturated fatty acids, which can reduce the contents of TG and TC in the blood and increase the content of HDL-C in the blood. At present, natural fish oil has been widely used in clinical practice as a lipid-lowering drug, which mainly inhibits the activity of hydroxymethylglutaryl coenzyme -A(HMG-CoA) reductase and reduces the synthesis of TC *in vivo*, while feeding back the up-regulation of LDL receptor level on the surface of hepatocytes to eliminate plasma LDL. However, it should be noted that in people with acute pancreatitis, high concentrations of USFA can cause damage to acinar cells and promote the development of pancreatitis. USFA may play a unique role in the pathogenesis of pancreatitis by activating PKC family members [22].

3. Foods rich in polysaccharides have attracted much attention due to their lipid-regulating activity, with fungal polysaccharides as the major ones, such as Ganoderma, *Lentinus edodes*, Auricularia, *Grifola frondosa*, Russula, Monascus, Poria, Cordyceps, *Agaricus blazei*, Tremella, *Dictyophora indusiata*, *Coriolus versicolor*, *Cordyceps militaris*, *Armillaria mellea*, *Pleurotus ostreatus*, and *Flammulina velutipes*. *Ganoderma lucidum* is taken as an example. Modern medical pharmacology research and clinical application have proved that *Ganoderma lucidum* not only has the functions of delaying aging, improving immunity and anti-inflammation, but also has the efficacy of reducing total cholesterol and regulating blood lipids [23]. Studies have shown that *Ganoderma lucidum* polysaccharides (GLP) and alkaloids contained in *Ganoderma lucidum* are the main active components that play a role in the regulation of blood lipids, and can play a role in reducing serum TG and TC [24]. As for the mechanism, it is currently more considered that GLP may reduce the synthesis of TC and TG *in vivo* by inhibiting the expression of key enzymes in the lipid synthesis pathway. In cell experiments, GLP was found to inhibit the mRNA expression of hydroxymethyl glutaryl coenzyme -A(HMG-CoA) reductase and fatty acid synthase (FAS) in HepG2 cells [25]. In addition to Ganoderma, other edible fungi are also rich in a variety of polysaccharides, such as lentinan, *Auricularia auricula* polysaccharide, have a certain effect on the regulation of blood lipids. Therefore, eating foods rich in polysaccharides is a very healthy dietary choice and an effective method for preventing and treating hyperlipidemia.

4. Foods containing polyphenol compounds have attracted much attention in the development of antioxidant health products. Polyphenols play an important role in increasing the levels of HDL and adiponectin, and preventing the oxidation of LDL. Common polyphenol compounds include anthocyanin, grape seed oil, astaxanthin, and lutein. Cinnamon is rich in polyphenols, which can activate transcription factors and antioxidant defense signaling pathways in the liver to reduce hyperlipidemia, inflammation, and oxidative stress [26].

Previous studies have shown that in France and some countries and regions with high wine consumption, even if people have the habit of high-fat diet, the incidence of cardiovascular disease is not high. This may be due to the antioxidant activity of polyphenols in wine and their effect in reducing total cholesterol absorption by increasing bile acids divided by. Gamboge is a plant growing in northeastern India. Its fruit is rich in polyphenols. Studies have shown that the fruit extract of this plant has a positive role in the prevention of hyperlipidemia [27]. In addition to food, drinking tea can also prevent hyperlipidemia and its concurrent diseases [28]. Tea is rich in catecholamine-based tea polyphenols. The current research has shown that tea polyphenols can improve the level of HDL-C and lecithin-cholesterol acyltransferase (LCAT) activity, and inhibit the intestinal absorption of exogenous TC, inhibit the activity of eugenol epoxidase to reduce TC biosynthesis, up-regulate LDL receptor level, reduce the secretion of apolipoprotein B100(ApoB100), accelerate TC transformation, and promote TC excretion to regulate TC metabolism. On the other hand, tea polyphenols reduced the absorption of exogenous TG and the activity of FAS by inhibiting the activity of pancreatic lipase to reduce fatty acid synthesis. At the same time, tea polyphenols regulate TG metabolism by accelerating the conversion of TG and promoting the excretion of fatty acids. Foods and drinks containing polyphenols are a very healthy dietary choice and an effective way to prevent and treat hyperlipidemia and its related conditions.

5. Foods containing flavonoids and isoflavones have strong activity in the prevention and treatment of hyperlipidemia. Many studies reported the lipid-lowering effect of total flavonoid extracts from plants. Hawthorn leaves and fruits are high flavonoid content of food. Animal experiments showed that flavonoids could significantly reduce the levels of TC, TG, and LDL-C in hyperlipidemia rats, and played a significant role in the regulation of lipid metabolism in hyperlipidemia rats to improve their disorders. In a study on oat flavonoids, the researchers focused on the intestinal flora and showed that oat flavonoids had anti-hyperlipidemia effect by interfering with bile acid metabolism and intestinal microflora [14]. In addition, the effect of flavonoids on reducing blood lipid was closely related to the number of free methylations. Studies have shown that the more methylation, the stronger the effect of flavonoids in reducing blood lipid. Isoflavones were corresponding to flavonoids. The main active components of soybean isoflavones were free aglycones genistein (Gen) and daidzein (Den). Similarly, soy isoflavones also reduced TC, TG, and LDL-C levels in hyperlipidemia, although its effect is not obvious [29].

6. Vitamin plays an important role in lipid metabolism. Among them, the effect of vitamin D is the most significant [30]. Vitamin D can reduce the acetylation or oxidation of LDL-C and inhibit the absorption of acetylated and oxidized LDL by macrophages to reduce the formation of foam cells and inhibit the formation of plaques. However, it should be noted that vitamin D is a double-edged sword for vascular calcification. Excessive or lack of vitamin D can lead to vascular calcification. Vitamin E is an important antioxidant in the body. Although the mechanism of its regulatory effect on blood lipid is not clear, hyperlipidemia has been determined to be inhibited by high vitamin E intake at animal levels. In addition to the antioxidant effect of vitamin E, vitamins A and C also have a certain

antioxidant capacity, which can be used as an auxiliary prevention and treatment strategy of hyperlipidemia.

In conclusion, prevention and adjuvant treatment of hyperlipidemia are extremely important by reducing the intake of cholesterol and saturated fatty acids, supplemented by a diet that reduces blood lipids.

3. The effect and improvement of exercise on hyperlipidemia

3.1 Mechanism of action of insufficient exercise on dyslipidemia

Studies have shown that good regular exercise can activate LPL in skeletal muscle and fat cells, promote the balanced transfer of VLDL and HDL-C, reduce serum TC, TG, and LDL, and increase HDL-C levels. Lack of exercise leads to a decrease in triglycerides depleted, an increase in endogenous triglyceride synthesis; moreover, it reduces LPL activity, slowing down triglyceride clearance which is especially common in the elderly [1]. When there is a lack of exercise, the secretion of epinephrine and norepinephrine decreases, and reduces the activity of LPL and the decomposition of fat in adipose tissue. At the same time, if the secretion of adrenaline and norepinephrine decreases, it may lead to the decrease of lipolysis, and at the same time, the activity of lipoxygenase increases, leading to the increase in fat synthesis. It is well known that short-term high-intensity exercise is mainly powered by sugar, while moderate-intensity long-term exercise is mainly powered by fat. During exercise, the body increases the call to triglycerides, muscles will enhance the intake of free fatty acids in the blood, and lack of exercise will lead to a decrease in mobilized triglycerides, thereby reducing the appearance of free fatty acids in the blood, also leading to a decrease in the intake of free fatty acids in the blood by muscles. At the same time, it should be noted that high triglyceride levels promote the occurrence of other metabolic disorders such as diabetes and CVD [31]. A lack of muscle exercise can impair glucose utilization, leading to the conversion of excess glucose into fat and increasing fat formation and accumulation in the blood. Regular exercise can improve insulin sensitivity and glucose uptake in muscles, which can help to prevent the conversion of excess glucose into fat and reduce the amount of fat in the blood. In general, exercise is extremely important for the prevention of CVD, and the lack of exercise increases the incidence of cardiovascular disease [32]. At the same time, as a way to prevent CVD and treat diabetes, the role played by exercise training should not be ignored [33].

In addition to the traditional mechanisms described above, other studies have revealed mechanisms by which lack of exercise alters lipid profile. Lack of exercise leads to less TG consumed by muscle tissue and a decrease in LPL, resulting in less TG hydrolysis. More subtilisin-invertase 9 (PCSK9) allows the liver to absorb and excrete less LDL, thereby increasing the amount of lipids in the blood.

3.2 Physical manifestations of hyperlipidemia caused by exercise

Hyperlipidemia is when blood levels of lipids such as cholesterol and triglycerides are higher than normal, which can lead to health problems such as heart disease and stroke. Exercise is an effective way to lower blood lipid levels, but if exercise is excessive or inappropriate, it can also lead to some physiological problems.

Hyperlipidemia caused by exercise is mainly manifested in the following aspects: (1) Muscle damage: Excessive exercise can cause muscle damage, releasing substances such as myoglobin and creatine kinase, which can affect liver function and lead to elevated cholesterol levels. (2) Muscle fatigue: Excessive exercise can fatigue muscles, which affects the oxidative metabolism of fatty acids, allowing fat to accumulate in the body, resulting in elevated blood lipid levels. (3) Active problems: Excessive exercise may lead to digestive disorders such as gastrointestinal discomfort and diarrhea, which may affect the absorption and metabolism of fat. (4) Hydration status: Excessive exercise may lead to dehydration, which may affect the concentration and metabolism of lipids in the blood.

Therefore, it is necessary to pay attention to the reasonable control of the amount of exercise to avoid hyperlipidemia caused by excessive exercise. In addition, it is necessary to combine diet, lifestyle, and other factors to comprehensively reduce blood lipid levels to maintain good health.

3.3 Improvement effect of different exercise methods and exercise intensity on hyperlipidemia

Previous studies have shown that exercise training can improve blood lipids, although to a limited extent. Different exercise methods and exercise intensity hyperlipidemia bring different improvements, the following will take specific studies as an example to explain the effects of different exercise modes and exercise intensity on blood lipid changes.

1. Aerobic exercise. Aerobic exercise is the most common and popular form of exercise. Aerobic exercise is defined as any form of physical activity that raises heart rate and breathing volume to meet the oxygen needs of the muscles that activate. Aerobic exercise is easier to perform than medication and has fewer side effects. Experiments have shown that aerobic exercise can significantly reduce blood lipids and increase HDL-C [34]. Several studies have further analyzed the effects of different aerobic exercise intensity and duration on lipids. For example, Kraus et al. randomized 111 overweight patients with mild-to-moderate dyslipidemia and sedentary habits into a control group and three aerobic training groups: high-intensity/high-activity aerobic exercise, high-intensity/low-exercise aerobic exercise, and moderate-intensity/low-exercise aerobic exercise. The results showed that the blood lipid changes in the high total exercise group and the high-intensity group were significantly better than those in the low total exercise group and the control group. The improvement in lipid levels in the low total exercise group was better than in the control group [35]. These findings indicate that overall aerobic exercise has a greater impact on blood lipid levels compared to the intensity of exercise. Within a certain range of exercise intensity, increasing exercise intensity can enhance the beneficial effects on blood lipids, but beyond a certain point, the positive effects of exercise on blood lipids tend to diminish. For instance, research has shown that low-intensity exercise can improve lipoprotein cholesterol compared to short-term high-intensity exercise [36].

2. Resistance training, also known as strength training. Studies have shown that strength training of a certain intensity can also significantly reduce blood lipid levels in the body. For example, a prospective study of lipid and lipoprotein levels in previously sedentary men (mean age 33) and women undergoing 16 weeks

of weight training (mean age 27) found that after 16 weeks of strength training, women reduced cholesterol by 9.5%, LDL-C by 17.9%, and triglycerides by 28.3%. The ratio of total HDL-C and low-density lipoprotein cholesterol-high lipoprotein cholesterol decreased by 14.3% and 20.3%, respectively. In men, LDL-C was reduced by 16.2 percent, while the proportion of total HDL-C and LDL-C decreased by 21.6 and 28.9%, respectively [37].

3. Effects of aerobic training in combination with other training on lipids. The combination of strength training and aerobic training can improve lipid metabolism by increasing the activity of key enzymes and promoting the breakdown and excretion of fats and cholesterol. This can lead to improvements in cardiovascular health and a reduced risk of metabolic diseases such as hyperlipidemia and atherosclerosis. Strength training combined with aerobic training can better promote the secretion of lipolytic hormone in the body and reduce insulin secretion. It not only increases fat mobilization and burning, but also increases the gene expression level of high-density lipoprotein receptor, increases the induction synthesis of HDL-C-related APOA1 apolipoprotein, increases the level of HDL-C in the body, and also reduces the level of LDL-C in the blood, so that the body can improve the metabolic capacity of cholesterol and cholesterol esters, and achieve the purpose of reducing blood lipids.

In addition to the above-mentioned exercise, Tai Ji Chuan in the prevention and improvement of hyperlipidemia has been studied, the study shows that Tai Ji Chuan in the promotion of whole body blood lectured, regulating blood lipids in the human body, etc. [38]. Brisk walking is very popular among middle-aged and elderly people, while patients with hyperlipidemia can choose the exercise time and intensity according to their own situation to achieve the purpose of alleviating hyperlipidemia.

3.4 Establish reasonable exercise habits

There is no doubt that exercise has a clear regulatory effect on blood lipids, and numerous studies have shown that exercise not only has a positive effect on dyslipidemia patients, but also helps to improve blood lipid status. However, there are many things to be aware of before starting to exercise. The most important thing is to choose the right exercise method for your physical condition and make a reasonable exercise plan. Reasonable exercise habits can help you better reduce blood lipids, improve dyslipidemia, and maintain health.

1. Be sure to warm up before exercise, warming up can improve the excitability of the central nervous system and muscles—awaken all parts of the human body involved in movement, and improve the excitability of the neuromuscular system. Improve muscle blood supply, activate muscle fibers, accelerate the contraction and relaxation of active muscles and antagonist muscles, produce a post-activation enhancement effect, and increase the contraction speed and contraction force of muscles, and be more conducive to exercise [39]. After warming up and raising body temperature, the elasticity and stretch ability of muscles and ligaments increases, so that muscle viscosity decreases, elasticity is enhanced, and the probability of sports injuries is reduced, and at the same time, by increasing body temperature, accelerating the speed of energy supply to the body, strengthening the metabolic process of substances in the body, it can also consume more fat and better reduce blood lipids.

2. Reasonably plan your exercise intensity and exercise time. Too high or too low exercise intensity is not conducive to causing significant improvement in blood lipids. Most of the beneficial changes occur when the intensity of exercise training is between 50 and 70% of the maximum oxygen uptake, and high-intensity exercise training does not appear to bring more beneficial changes than moderate- and low-intensity exercise training. Animal experiments have also confirmed that too high-intensity endurance exercise training not only does not improve dyslipidemia, but may accelerate the occurrence of dyslipidemia. Therefore, too intense exercise intensity or too long exercise is not suitable. The intensity of exercise is best at moderate intensity and is not recommended to exceed it. The test is based on your heart rate per minute to judge your exercise intensity. The target heart rate value is calculated as: [220-age (1 year old)] × 60–70%, which is the moderate-intensity exercise range, and be sure to use the heart rate intensity range that you can accept. In terms of exercise time, exercise for at least 30 minutes a day, and 60 minutes is better. If it is difficult to exercise for 30 minutes at a time, start with 10 minutes and accumulate through multiple 10 minutes to 30 minutes. LDL is the largest part of total cholesterol, this reflects changes in total cholesterol levels. For people who want to improve hyperlipidemia, lowering higher LDL indicators is the most important goal. This requires at least 250–300 minutes of aerobic exercise per week, burning about 2000 kilocalories to help reduce fat content and body weight, and is expected to reduce LDL-C by about 5–8% after 12–16 weeks.

4. The influence and regulation of psychological factors on hyperlipidemia

4.1 Mechanism of action of psycho-emotional state on lipid metabolism

Usually, when a person is in a stable emotional state, the lipid metabolism process does not undergo significant changes. The metabolism of triglycerides, phospholipids, cholesterol, and plasma lipoproteins is regulated by insulin, glucagon, diet, nutrition, biochemical enzyme activity in the body, and other complex and precise regulations, and is transformed into material components required for various fine biochemical reactions in the body. The liver, adipose tissue, and small intestine are important sites for synthesizing fat, with the liver having the strongest synthesis ability. After synthesis, it needs to combine with apolipoprotein, cholesterol, etc., to form extremely LDL, which is transported into the bloodstream and stored or utilized in extrahepatic tissues.

When psychological stress occurs, lipid metabolism changes accordingly, and psychological stress includes two types: chronic and acute. Previous studies have shown that acute psychological stress has a relatively small impact on blood lipids, while chronic psychological stress may have a more significant impact on the occurrence and development of CVD. The mode of action of acute psychological stress is relatively strong and one time; chronic psychological stress is relatively mild, but it occurs frequently and lasts for a long time, usually from days to months. At present, the mechanism by which stress causes an increase in plasma lipid concentration is still unclear. One viewpoint is to use a stress-induced lipolysis model to explain the increase in blood lipids, which refers to an increase in cholesterol secretion by the liver during the stress process, leading to an increase in circulating cholesterol concentration. Adrenaline affects the activity of lipoprotein lipase, liver lipase, and other hormone-sensitive lipases, thereby increasing the release of fatty acids from adipose tissue and providing the liver with substrates for the synthesis of TG and VLDL. *In vitro* experiments have shown that adrenaline can effectively inhibit the secretion of lipoprotein lipase and human leukocyte antigen after translation. In addition, adrenaline may directly stimulate the release of free fatty acids in adipose tissue, which accelerates the process of liver cholesterol secretion.

4.2 Interaction between dyslipidemia and mental state

The psychological risk factors of patients with hyperlipidemia include somatization, interpersonal disorders, marital discord, anxiety, depression, and anger. At the same time, it was also found that the psychological risk factors of hyperlipidemia patients include age, educational level, gender, lifestyle habits, dietary structure, body mass index, and potential social discrimination. Patients with long-term hyperlipidemia often also suffer from diseases such as coronary heart disease and pancreatitis. These diseases can bring great mental pressure to patients, leading to extreme emotions such as anxiety and anger. Under the influence of extreme emotions, physical and mental health can face great threats. Emotional regulation plays an important role in alleviating the negative impact of dyslipidemia on mental state. Type 2 diabetes mellitus (T2DM) can cause secondary hyperlipidemia. Patients with type 2 diabetes treated with insulin typically have more comorbidities [40]. Emotional distress was the most common type of distress in T2DM patients using antihypertensive or antihyperlipidemic medications [41]. High blood lipids can also cause other diseases, and hypercholesterolemia are possible risk factors for restless leg syndrome [42]. Dyslipidemia is the main cause of cardiovascular complications in diabetes mellitus (DM) [43].

Different people have different psychological resilience, pressure resistance, and perception of the external environment, so the way they handle negative emotions also varies. Some people are very sensitive, while others are not easily influenced. Faced with the generation of negative emotions, a group of people usually resort to the bad practice of overeating. Impulsive behavior when distressed exacerbated the link between weight-based teasing distress and loss of control eating frequency [44]. Overweight patients should be informed that there is not only a risk for the commonly known consequences such as diabetes, hypertension, coronary artery disease, and heart failure, but also that there is a greater risk of developing atrial fibrillation and a subsequent risk of stroke and death [45]. This usually leads to a sudden increase in obesity and a surge in body mass index. There is a close relationship between body mass index and hyperlipidemia patients, and the higher the body mass index, the higher the incidence rate. Obese people accumulate a large amount of fat in their bodies, which leads to the accumulation of triglycerides in the liver endoplasmic reticulum. They cannot combine extremely dense lipoprotein to secrete into the blood circulation, which leads to the disorder of fat metabolism and the increase of blood lipids.

To alleviate the mental stress caused by dyslipidemia, patients should avoid emotional tension and excessive excitement, which can cause an increase in blood cholesterol and triglycerides levels. In such cases, small doses of sedatives can be used, to avoid mental side effects caused by long-term medication use by patients.

4.3 How to maintain a good mood

Current guidelines do not stipulate the atherogenic lipid profile in the postprandial state as a target for therapy nor do they give any target values for the parameters of postprandial hyperlipidemia [46]. Therefore, maintaining a good emotional state is necessary for physical and mental health, and the following activities can be used to maintain a good mood. Some people choose to use prayer to maintain stable emotions. We did not find a significant association between the perceived appropriateness of one's emotional reaction and use of prayer to manage emotions [47]. You can go to a hair salon to get a new hairstyle. Psychologists believe that if a person change their hairstyle when their mood goes bad, it can suppress the early onset of bad emotions and interfere with the production of hormones that cause depression. Moreover, changing hairstyles can provide psychological relaxation and pleasure, leading to an improvement in mood. Limited social competence hinders acquisition of adequate coping strategies [48]. A balanced diet is also important for maintaining health and maintaining a healthy mindset. Firstly, add sweet potatoes or yams to rice. Secondly, it is important to eat more leafy vegetables and add nuts to the dishes. Crushed nuts can not only be seasoned, but also reduce the use of salt. The third is that appropriate seaweed can be added to the soup.

The improvement of mood through exercise cannot be ignored. Individual responses to anger reduction are idiosyncratic and the match between the individual and the activity may be more crucial than the activity itself [49]. Regular and moderate exercise can help us overcome symptoms of depression and anger. Compared to using medication, exercise can alleviate stress caused by lipid abnormalities. Exercise can alleviate anxiety. Anxiety is another extremely common emotional disorder, manifested in a loss of interest in life and fear of bad outcomes, helping people restore inner peace and relaxation. Through the continuous accumulation of exercise, people will also gain higher self-esteem and increased confidence through self-transcendence. We can also do more mental health tests in our daily lives to ensure that our emotional state is in a relatively positive state, in order to make timely adjustments. But remember, whatever the mechanism, it will be important to determine whether mental stress testing provides additional risk prediction above and beyond the other traditional risk stratification tools in different categories of patients [50].

5. The impact and prevention of risk factors on hyperlipidemia

5.1 Close relationship between bad lifestyle habits and hyperlipidemia

Studies have shown that smoking, alcohol consumption, lack of physical activity, and low intake of vegetables and fruits are positively associated with dyslipidemia [51].

The rate of dyslipidemia in smokers is significantly higher than in non-smokers. This is because the nicotine and carbon monoxide contained in tobacco can increase oxidative modification, enhance platelet agglomeration, increase the content of TG, TC and LDL-C in the body, and reduce the content of HDL-C [52]. Smoking can affect blood lipid metabolism, and long-term smoking will promote platelet aggregation and coronary thrombosis, lead to a decrease in vascular endothelial progenitor cells, slow down the new generation of micro-vessels, and damage to large blood vessel repair [53]. At the same time, it leads to oxidative stress and inflammatory response, so that the coagulation fibrinolytic system in the body is dysfunctional. Moreover, it affects blood lipid metabolism, and induces or aggravates atherosclerosis and coronary artery spasm. The TC level of smokers was positively correlated with the age of cigarettes smoked and the number of cigarettes smoked, while the HDL-C level was negatively correlated with it. The greater the amount smoked by smokers, the higher the total cholesterol, total triglycerides, TC/HDL, apolipoprotein, and LDL, which were significantly higher than those who smoked a small amount and did not smoke. Its HDL and apolipoprotein are significantly lower than those who smoke a small amount and those who do not smoke. The rate of dyslipidemia in people who drink too much is significantly higher than in those who drink little or non-alcohol [54]. Since alcohol can increase the mobilization of peripheral adipose tissue in the human body, increase the synthesis of triacylglycerol in the liver, and reduce the oxidation of fatty acids, resulting in hyperlipidemia, the higher the amount of alcohol intake, the higher the incidence of dyslipidemia. Long-term heavy drinking can lead to alcoholic liver disease [55], which initially manifests as fatty liver. Patients with alcoholic liver disease have poor liver reserve and lipid levels decrease significantly as the disease progresses. In patients with alcoholic fatty liver disease, blood lipids are increased, and triglycerides are more pronounced. The patient's liver function level will decrease with the degree of decompensation of cirrhosis, and the blood lipid TG and TC levels will also decrease. Alcoholic liver disease severely affects lipid metabolism, so changes in liver function are often accompanied by changes in lipids.

In addition, the risk of chronic diseases may be higher in people who regularly eat smoked bacon compared to those who do not eat smoked bacon. The risk of chronic diseases may also be higher in people who frequently eat out or socialize compared to those who do not or only occasionally do so. On the other hand, people who consume moderate amounts of meat may have a lower risk of chronic diseases compared to those who eat a lot of meat. Bad lifestyle habits are an important influencing factor in the development of chronic diseases. However, the prevention of chronic diseases is a complex issue that involves multiple factors in their pathogenesis.

5.2 How to reduce the risk of risk factors for dyslipidemia

Dyslipidemia is easily overlooked because it is not accompanied by obvious clinical manifestations, but the various diseases caused by it can seriously affect the quality of people's life. Current research suggests that dyslipidemia's mechanisms are closely related and interconnected, and co-occurring chronic diseases are common. However, many potential mechanisms of action still need to be explored further. The interaction of multiple chronic diseases can pose greater health hazards to the population than single-disease chronic diseases [56]. For people with high-risk factors, effective prevention and treatment measures can help reduce the risk of dyslipidemia and its associated health risks. It is particularly important to prevent the occurrence of chronic diseases, especially chronic comorbidities.

We should focus on the lipid levels of patients with hypertension, diabetes, and hyperuricemia, especially in donors who are closely related to cardiovascular disease, to prevent the occurrence of cardiovascular disease. It is suggested that relevant departments should incorporate school testing into the free routine physical examination items for residents when formulating health prevention strategies and measures, use community resources to advocate a healthy lifestyle, adopt comprehensive measures such as scientific diet, reasonable nutrition, smoking cessation and alcohol abstinence [57], recompose sleep, control weight, strengthen exercise, and control blood sugar of diabetic patients to reduce blood lipid levels, and reduce the prevalence of dyslipidemia and the prevalence of chronic diseases. Try to achieve early detection and early treatment of chronic diseases, reduce the occurrence of complications and disabilities, reduce the pain of patients, and improve the health level of patients. High-risk groups and patients need to understand diseases, standardize behavior and lifestyle, reduce risk factors, improve the awareness, treatment, and control rates of high-risk groups with dyslipidemia, correct bad living habits, and better grasp disease prevention and prevention measures [58].

Lifestyle therapy is the core strategy of dyslipidemia management, and strengthening health awareness and awareness of related disease risks, developing healthy lifestyle, and eating habits have become the key to prevention and treatment. Therefore, residents can adopt some measures in their lifestyle to reduce the risk of dyslipidemia risk factors, such as low-carbohydrate diet and Mediterranean diet [59], actively improve dietary nutritional structure [60, 61], and at the same time carry out appropriate activities to prevent calorie accumulation [62]. These measures were all associated with reduced TG levels and elevated HDL-C levels. Among them, exercise can significantly increase HDL-C and improve TG levels, reduce dietary animal fat intake, and can reduce the prevalence of blood lipids.

6. Conclusions

This chapter describes the causative mechanisms of hyperlipidemia and how to prevent it from several aspects: diet, exercise, psychological factors, and lifestyle risk factors. The descriptions provide the reader with a better understanding of the importance of lifestyle interventions for improving and preventing hyperlipidemia on a daily basis. After the development of hyperlipidemia, it is even more important to strengthen and pay attention to the aforementioned aspects in daily life. Attention should be paid to actively adopting various lifestyle interventions, which can restore the body to a healthy condition.

Notes/thanks/other declarations

This study was funded by Liaoning Province Applied Basic Research Program [grant number 2023JH2/101300098].

Author details

Shan Gao[1] and Zuowei Pei[1,2,3]*

1 Department of Central Laboratory, Central Hospital of Dalian University of Technology, Dalian, China

2 Department of Cardiology, Central Hospital of Dalian University of Technology, Dalian, China

3 Faculty of Medicine, Dalian University of Technology, Dalian, China

*Address all correspondence to: pzw_dl@163.com

References

[1] Karr S. Epidemiology and management of hyperlipidemia. The American Journal of Managed Care. 2017;**23**(9 Suppl.):S139-S148

[2] Berberich AJ, Hegele RA. A modern approach to dyslipidemia. Endocrine Reviews. 2022;**43**(4):611-653. DOI: 10.1210/endrev/bnab037

[3] Writing Group Members, Mozaffarian D, Benjamin EJ, et al. Heart disease and stroke Statistics-2016 update: A report from the American Heart Association [published correction appears in Circulation. 2016;133(15):e599]. Circulation. 2016;**133**(4):e38-e360. DOI: 10.1161/CIR.0000000000000350

[4] Parhofer KG, Laufs U. The diagnosis and treatment of hypertriglyceridemia. Deutsches Ärzteblatt International. 2019;**116**(49):825-832. DOI: 10.3238/arztebl.2019.0825

[5] Zhang QL, Wang Y, Liu JS, Du YZ. Effects of hypercaloric diet-induced hyperinsulinemia and hyperlipidemia on the ovarian follicular development in mice. The Journal of Reproduction and Development. 2022;**68**(3):173-180. DOI: 10.1262/jrd.2021-132

[6] Zhao S, Zhong J, Sun C, Zhang J. Effects of aerobic exercise on TC, HDL-C, LDL-C and TG in patients with hyperlipidemia: A protocol of systematic review and meta-analysis. Medicine (Baltimore). 2021;**100**(10):e25103. DOI: 10.1097/MD.0000000000025103

[7] Ghaemi SN, Shields GS, Hegarty JD, Goodwin FK. Cholesterol levels in mood disorders: High or low? Bipolar Disorders. 2000;**2**(1):60-64. DOI: 10.1034/j.1399-5618.2000.020109.x

[8] Leroux C, Brazeau AS, Gingras V, Desjardins K, Strychar I, Rabasa-Lhoret R. Lifestyle and cardiometabolic risk in adults with type 1 diabetes: A review. Canadian Journal of Diabetes. 2014;**38**(1):62-69. DOI: 10.1016/j.jcjd.2013.08.268

[9] Yan H, Niimi M, Matsuhisa F, et al. Apolipoprotein CIII deficiency protects against atherosclerosis in knockout rabbits. Arteriosclerosis, Thrombosis, and Vascular Biology. 2020;**40**(9):2095-2107. DOI: 10.1161/ATVBAHA.120.314368

[10] Mach F, Baigent C, Catapano AL, et al. 2019 ESC/EAS guidelines for the management of dyslipidaemias: Lipid modification to reduce cardiovascular risk, [published correction appears in Eur Heart J. 2020 Nov 21;41(44):4255]. European Heart Journal. 2020;**41**(1):111-188. DOI: 10.1093/eurheartj/ehz455

[11] Estruch R, Ros E, Salas-Salvadó J, et al. Primary prevention of cardiovascular disease with a Mediterranean diet supplemented with extra-virgin olive oil or nuts. The New England Journal of Medicine. 2018;**378**(25):e34. DOI: 10.1056/NEJMoa1800389

[12] Marra F, Svegliati-Baroni G. Lipotoxicity and the gut-liver axis in NASH pathogenesis. Journal of Hepatology. 2018;**68**(2):280-295. DOI: 10.1016/j.jhep.2017.11.014

[13] Hill MF, Bordoni B. Hyperlipidemia [Internet]. Treasure Island (FL): StatPearls Publishing; 2023

[14] Duan R, Guan X, Huang K, et al. Flavonoids from whole-grain oat alleviated high-fat diet-induced

hyperlipidemia via regulating bile acid metabolism and gut microbiota in mice. Journal of Agricultural and Food Chemistry. 2021;**69**(27):7629-7640. DOI: 10.1021/acs.jafc.1c01813

[15] McCrindle BW. Hyperlipidemia in children. Thrombosis Research. 2006;**118**(1):49-58. DOI: 10.1016/j.thromres.2005.01.006

[16] Nie Y, Luo F. Dietary fiber: An opportunity for a global control of hyperlipidemia. Oxidative Medicine and Cellular Longevity. 2021;**2021**:5542342. Published 2021 Apr 8. DOI: 10.1155/2021/5542342

[17] O'Grady J, O'Connor EM, Shanahan F. Review article: Dietary fibre in the era of microbiome science. Alimentary Pharmacology & Therapeutics. 2019;**49**(5):506-515. DOI: 10.1111/apt.15129

[18] O'Keefe SJ. The association between dietary fibre deficiency and high-income lifestyle-associated diseases: Burkitt's hypothesis revisited. The Lancet Gastroenterology & Hepatology. 2019;**4**(12):984-996. DOI: 10.1016/S2468-1253(19)30257-2

[19] Ozyurt VH, Ötles S. Effect of food processing on the physicochemical properties of dietary fibre. Acta Scientiarum Polonorum. Technologia Alimentaria. 2016;**15**(3):233-245. DOI: 10.17306/J.AFS.2016.3.23

[20] Junejo SA, Zhang L, Yang L, et al. Anti-hyperlipidemic and hepatoprotective properties of wheat bran with different particle sizes. Journal of the Science of Food and Agriculture. 2019;**99**(4):1990-1996. DOI: 10.1002/jsfa.9397

[21] Yang Y, Ge S, Chen Q, et al. Chlorella unsaturated fatty acids suppress high-fat diet-induced obesity in C57/BL6J mice. Journal of Food Science. 2022;**87**(8):3644-3658. DOI: 10.1111/1750-3841.16246

[22] Chang YT, Chang MC, Tung CC, Wei SC, Wong JM. Distinctive roles of unsaturated and saturated fatty acids in hyperlipidemic pancreatitis. World Journal of Gastroenterology. 2015;**21**(32):9534-9543. DOI: 10.3748/wjg.v21.i32.9534

[23] Sang T, Guo C, Guo D, et al. Suppression of obesity and inflammation by polysaccharide from sporoderm-broken spore of *Ganoderma lucidum* via gut microbiota regulation. Carbohydrate Polymers. 2021;**256**:117594. DOI: 10.1016/j.carbpol.2020.117594

[24] Wu S. Hypolipidaemic and anti-lipidperoxidant activities of *Ganoderma lucidum* polysaccharide. International Journal of Biological Macromolecules. 2018;**118**(Pt B):2001-2005. DOI: 10.1016/j.ijbiomac.2018.07.082

[25] Yang M, Hu D, Cui Z, Li H, Man C, Jiang Y. Lipid-lowering effects of *Inonotus obliquus* polysaccharide *in vivo* and *in vitro*. Food. 2021;**10**(12):3085. Published 2021 Dec 12. DOI: 10.3390/foods10123085

[26] Tuzcu Z, Orhan C, Sahin N, Juturu V, Sahin K. Cinnamon polyphenol extract inhibits hyperlipidemia and inflammation by modulation of transcription factors in high-fat diet-fed rats. Oxidative Medicine and Cellular Longevity. 2017;**2017**:1583098. DOI: 10.1155/2017/1583098

[27] Sarma R, Kumari S, Elancheran R, Deori M, Devi R. Polyphenol rich extract of *Garcinia pedunculata* fruit attenuates the hyperlipidemia induced by high fat diet. Frontiers in Pharmacology. 2016;**7**:294. Published 2016 Aug 31. DOI: 10.3389/fphar.2016.00294

[28] Ishida N, Iizuka M, Kataoka K, et al. Improvement of blood lipid profiles by Goishi tea polyphenols in a randomised, double-blind, placebo-controlled clinical study. International Journal of Food Sciences and Nutrition. 2018;**69**(5):598-607. DOI: 10.1080/09637486.2017.1386629

[29] Qin Y, Niu K, Zeng Y, et al. Isoflavones for hypercholesterolaemia in adults. Cochrane Database of Systematic Reviews. 2013;**6**:CD009518. Published 2013 Jun 6. DOI: 10.1002/14651858.CD009518.pub2

[30] Zhang W, Yi J, Liu D, et al. The effect of vitamin D on the lipid profile as a risk factor for coronary heart disease in postmenopausal women: A meta-analysis and systematic review of randomized controlled trials. Experimental Gerontology. 2022;**161**:111709. DOI: 10.1016/j.exger.2022.111709

[31] Jeppesen J, Hein HO, Suadicani P, Gyntelberg F. Triglyceride concentration and ischemic heart disease: An eight-year follow-up in the Copenhagen male study, [published correction appears in circulation 1998 may 19;97(19):1995]. Circulation. 1998;**97**(11):1029-1036. DOI: 10.1161/01.cir.97.11.1029

[32] Erlichman J, Kerbey AL, James WP. Physical activity and its impact on health outcomes. Paper 1: The impact of physical activity on cardiovascular disease and all-cause mortality: An historical perspective. Obesity Reviews. 2002;**3**(4):257-271. DOI: 10.1046/j.1467-789x.2002.00077.x

[33] Pearson TA, Blair SN, Daniels SR, et al. AHA guidelines for primary prevention of cardiovascular disease and stroke: 2002 update: Consensus panel guide to comprehensive risk reduction for adult patients without coronary or other atherosclerotic vascular diseases. American Heart Association science advisory and coordinating committee. Circulation. 2002;**106**(3):388-391. DOI: 10.1161/01.cir.0000020190.45892.75

[34] Kelley GA, Kelley KS. Aerobic exercise and lipids and lipoproteins in men: A meta-analysis of randomized controlled trials. The Journal of Men's Health & Gender. 2006;**3**(1):61-70. DOI: 10.1016/j.jmhg.2005.09.003

[35] Kraus WE, Houmard JA, Duscha BD, et al. Effects of the amount and intensity of exercise on plasma lipoproteins. The New England Journal of Medicine. 2002;**347**(19):1483-1492. DOI: 10.1056/NEJMoa020194

[36] He N, Ye H. Exercise and hyperlipidemia. Advances in Experimental Medicine and Biology. 2020;**1228**:79-90. DOI: 10.1007/978-981-15-1792-1_5

[37] Goldberg L, Elliot DL, Schutz RW, Kloster FE. Changes in lipid and lipoprotein levels after weight training. Journal of the American Medical Association. 1984;**252**(4):504-506

[38] Hui DS, Hall S, Chan MT, Joynt GM, Chow B, Sung JJ. Risks posed by the use of oxygen therapy and non-invasive positive pressure ventilation: A pilot study. Hong Kong Medical Journal. 2009;**15**(Suppl. 8):4-7

[39] Blazevich AJ, Gill ND, Kvorning T, et al. No effect of muscle stretching within a full, dynamic warm-up on athletic performance. Medicine and Science in Sports and Exercise. 2018;**50**(6):1258-1266. DOI: 10.1249/MSS.0000000000001539

[40] Gyldenkerne C, Olesen KKW, Madsen M, Thim T, Jensen LO,

Raungaard B, et al. Association between anti-diabetes treatments and cardiovascular risk in diabetes patients with and without coronary artery disease. Diabetes and Vascular Disease Research. 2019;**16**(4):351-359

[41] Alfian Sofa D, Nurul A, Aulia I, Perwitasari Dyah A, Petra D, Eelko H, et al. Emotional distress is associated with lower health-related quality of life among patients with diabetes using antihypertensive and/or Antihyperlipidemic medications: A multicenter study in Indonesia. Therapeutics and Clinical Risk Management. 2021;**17**:1333-1342

[42] Katerina DV, Yanping L, Salma B-A, Yi N, Jiali H, Xiang G. Prospective study of obesity, hypertension, high cholesterol, and risk of restless legs syndrome. Movement Disorders. 2014;**29**(8):1044-1052

[43] Sholhui P, Wookeun L, Sun CH, Sook HK. Diagnostic utility of serum glycated albumin for diabetes mellitus and its correlation with hyperlipidemia. Annals of Laboratory Medicine. 2016;**36**(4):306-312

[44] Osa ML, Lisa B, Giuliani NR, Kelly NR. Associations among weight-based teasing distress, impulsive emotion regulation, and loss of control eating in racially and ethnically diverse young men. Eating Behaviors. 2021;**43**:101543, (prepublish)

[45] Bulent G, Antonio P, Benjamin Emelia J, Giuseppe B, Crijns Harry J, Fogel Richard I, et al. European heart rhythm association (EHRA)/European Association of Cardiovascular Prevention and Rehabilitation (EACPR) position paper on how to prevent atrial fibrillation endorsed by the Heart Rhythm Society (HRS) and Asia Pacific Heart Rhythm Society (APHRS). Europace: European Pacing, Arrhythmias, and Cardiac Electrophysiology. 2017;**19**(2):190-225

[46] la Paz M-d, Sergio BB, Cardelo Magdalena P, Sergio L, Rocio A, Muriana Francisco JG. Olive oil and postprandial hyperlipidemia: Implications for atherosclerosis and metabolic syndrome. Food and Function. 2016;7(12):4734-4744

[47] Sharp S, Carr D. The use of prayer to manage anger: Do characteristics of the emotional experience matter? Review of Religious Research. 2017;**59**(4):557-574

[48] Hodel B, Brenner HD, Merlo MC, Teuber JF. Emotional management therapy in early psychosis. The British Journal of Psychiatry Supplement. 1998;**172**(33):128-133

[49] Ferguson CJ, Maguire R, Lemar S. Pick your poison: Choice of activity determines mood management following a stressful task. Journal of Aggression, Maltreatment and Trauma. 2018;**27**(3):332-346

[50] Hassan M, York KM, Li Q, Lucey DG, Fillingim RB, Sheps DS. Variability of myocardial ischemic responses to mental versus exercise or adenosine stress in patients with coronary artery disease. Journal of Nuclear Cardiology. 2008;**15**(4):518-525

[51] Lee I, Kim S, Kang H. Lifestyle risk factors and all-cause and cardiovascular disease mortality: Data from the Korean longitudinal study of aging. International Journal of Environmental Research and Public Health. 2019;**10**:10260

[52] Shah J, Alsubaie ASR, Sehar B, et al. Association of cigarette smoking with hyperlipidemia in male individuals. Food and Nutrition Sciences. 2021;**12**(10):937-949. DOI: 10.4236/fns.2021.1210069

[53] Nakamura S, Kimura M, Goto C, et al. Cigarette smoking abolishes ischemic preconditioning-induced augmentation of endothelium-dependent vasodilation. Hypertension. 2009;**53**(4):674-681

[54] Oh SS, Kim W, Han KT, et al. Alcohol consumption frequency or alcohol intake per drinking session: Which has a larger impact on the metabolic syndrome and its components. Alcohol. 2018;**71**:15-23

[55] Shen Z, Li YM, Yu CH, et al. Risk factors for alcohol-related liver injury in the island population of China: A population-based case-control study. World Journal of Gastroenterology: WJG. 2008;**14**(14):2255

[56] Saligram N, Nugent R. Chronic diseases—The social justice issue of our time. The Lancet. 2016;**387**(10022):943

[57] Liu X, Peveri G, Bosetti C, Bagnardi V, Specchia C, Gallus S, et al. Dose-response relationships between cigarette smoking and kidney cancer: A systematic review and meta-analysis. Critical Reviews in Oncology/Hematology. 2019;**142**:86-93. DOI: 10.1016/j.critrevonc.2

[58] Olatona FA, Onabanjo OO, Ugbaja RN, et al. Dietary habits and metabolic risk factors for non-communicable diseases in a university undergraduate population. Journal of Health, Population, and Nutrition. 2018;**37**(1):21

[59] Kopel E, Sidi Y, Kivity S. Prevention of diabetes with Mediterranean diets. Annals of Internal Medicine. 2014;**161**(2):157

[60] He M, van Dam RM, Rimm E, et al. Whole-grain, cereal fiber, bran, and germ intake and the risks of all-cause and cardiovascular disease–specific mortality among women with type 2 diabetes mellitus. Circulation. 2010;**121**(20):2162-2168

[61] Burger KNJ, Beulens JWJ, van der Schouw YT, et al. Dietary fiber, carbohydrate quality and quantity, and mortality risk of individuals with diabetes mellitus. PLoS One. 2012;7(8):e43127

[62] Hu FB, Rimm EB, Stampfer MJ, et al. Prospective study of major dietary patterns and risk of coronary heart disease in men. The American Journal of Clinical Nutrition. 2000;**72**(4):912-921

Chapter 5

A New Algorithm for the Selection and Risk Stratification of Patients for the Efficient Aerobic Cardiorespiratory Training after Coronary Artery Bypass Surgery

Tea Kakuchaya, Leo Bockeria, Zarina Tokaeva, Nona Pachuashvili and Tamara Dzhitava

Abstract

The introduction of the strategically new algorithm for the preparing cardiac patients for aerobic exercise trainings of different intensity, with the transition from constant moderate-intensity training to high-intensity interval training, fundamentally changes medical approaches to cardiac rehabilitation after open heart surgery. We have developed such algorithms with the best combination of cardiovascular and non-cardiovascular parameters in patients after CABG.

Keywords: aerobic exercise training, coronary artery bypass surgery, risk stratification, exercise capacity, cardiovascular parameters, non-cardiovascular parameters

1. Introduction

In the recent past, patients who survived myocardial infarction were recommended bed rest for several weeks [1]. That was the common tactic. Currently, patients both after coronary artery stenting and after coronary artery bypass grafting are recommended aerobic physical trainings in complex postoperative treatment to improve functional capacity and reduce the risk of hospitalization and mortality [2].

It is of key importance to understand what the physiological mechanisms are that aerobic physical training influences the function of the cardiovascular system in patients with ischemic heart disease.

Randomized as well as non-randomized clinical trials, observational and case-control studies have proven that physical trainings significantly modify cardiovascular mortality risk and reduce major cardiovascular and cerebrovascular events [3, 4]. According to these studies overall mortality reduction has been beneficial in post-acute coronary syndrome and post-coronary artery bypass surgery (post-CABG) patients. The specific mechanisms by which physical activity

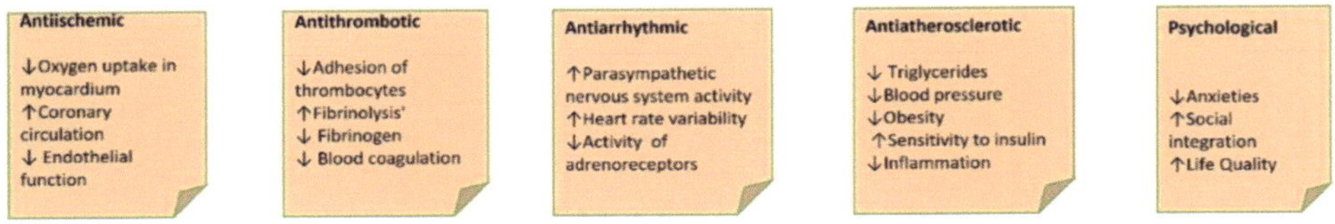

Figure 1.
Physiological and psychological effects of aerobic physical trainings in ischemic heart disease patients.

reduces mortality and cardiovascular complications are likely to be multifactorial and go beyond reducing cardiovascular disease (CVD) risk factors, as positive effects have also been observed on thrombosis, cardiac performance, cardiac remodeling, endothelial function, inflammation, and autonomic nervous system activity (**Figure 1**). It has been found that favorable impacts of exercise training on thrombotic modification are mediated by suppressed pro-thrombogenic factors and enhanced anti-thrombogenic factors [5]. Physical activity decreases exercise induced plasma catecholamine levels and down-regulates platelet α_2-adrenergic receptor performance, thereby reducing Von Willebrand factor-platelet interaction. Moreover, exercise training enhances substantial nitric oxide (NO) release from platelets and endothelium. Exercise training provides protection against oxidative stress by increasing NO bioavailability determining anti-hypertensive effects [6]. While managing oxidative stress exercise training facilitates reduction of systemic inflammatory markers. The increased content of mitochondria in muscles during exercise training promotes fat oxidation preferentially rather than carbohydrate oxidation. This adaptation reduces lactate production and provides longer training durations while increasing aerobic capacity. Improved cardiac performance mechanism lies through angiogenesis in muscle, mediated by B-adrenergic stimulation of capillary growth by vascular endothelial growth factors and platelet-derived growth factors. These processes are stimulated by insulin-like growth factor-1, proportionally expressed during exercise, and have been shown to reverse cardiac remodeling in animal models. Study by Soci UPR and co-authors [7] showed that post-transcriptional gene regulation associated with exercise training by microRNAs reduces remodeling through interactions between metabolic, contractile and epigenetic genes. Angiotensinogen II modulation during exercise training causes alterations in systemic vasoconstriction, sodium and water retention, and aldosterone production. Decreasing aldosterone lowers sympathetic tone. Another mechanism of regulating sympathetic tone is through the actions of plasma adrenomodullin [8] and atrio/brain-natriuretic-peptides which are tied closely to aerobic consumption [9]. These molecules attenuate blood pressure by suppressing noradrenaline and endothelin-1, improving endothelial responsiveness and function. Regular physical activity increases parasympathetic tone in sympathovagal signaling resulting in heart rate variability changes towards better prognosis.

A key requirement for the function of the cardiovascular system during exercise is to ensure the delivery of the necessary amount of oxygen and other nutrients to the working muscles. To this end, muscle blood flow during physical work increases tremendously [10]. The relationship between cardiac output and peripheral muscle function, and between oxygen consumption and peripheral muscle performance at different load levels, is linear. Muscle work increases the need for oxygen, and this,

Risk stratification (RR) protocols for CVD patients participating in cardiac rehabilitation (CR)				Reference
	Category of patients included	**Parameters used for RR**	**Risk groups**	
American Association of Cardiovascular and Pulmonary Rehabilitation (AACVPR)	Patients after MI, coronary revascularization	Stress-test with METs, ischemia, angina symptoms, silent ischemia, arrythmias, LV EF, BP, HR, CHF symptoms	Low, medium, high	[12]
American College of Sports Medicine (ACSM)	Patients with CVD and any other individuals	Stress-test with METs, ischemia, angina symptoms, silent ischemia, arrythmias, LV EF, BP, HR, CHF symptoms	Low, medium, high	[13]
American Heart Association (AHA)	Patients with various CVD, including congenital and acquired heart diseases, post-CABG, after stenting, chronic heart failure (CHF)	Stress-test with METs, ischemia, angina symptoms, arrythmias, LV EF, BP, CHF symptoms	Low, medium, high	[14]
F. Pashkow (USA)	Patients after MI, coronary revascularization	Stress-test with METs, perfusion and kinetical defects during stress tests, ischemia, angina symptoms, arrythmias, late ventricular potentials assessed by high resolution ECG, LV EF, BP, CHF symptoms	Low, medium, high	[15]
Brazilian Society of Cardiology (BSC)	Patients after MI, coronary revascularization	Stress-test with METs, ischemia, arrythmias, LV EF, BP, CHF symptoms	Low, medium, high	[16]
French Society of Cardiology (FSC)	Patients after MI, coronary revascularization	Stress-test with METs, ischemia, angina symptoms, arrythmias, LV EF, BP, CHF symptoms; echo- and ECG stress tests, anamnesis	Low, medium, high	[17]
Spanish Society of Cardiology (SSC)	Patients after MI, coronary revascularization	Stress-test with METs, stress-test with Thallium; ischemia, angina symptoms, arrythmias, LV EF, BP, CHF symptoms; $VO_{2\,max}$ for competitions	Low, medium, high	[18]

CVD—cardiovascular diseases; RR—risk stratification (risk of morbidity and mortality, associated with exercise trainings); MI—myocardial infarction, BP—blood pressure, HR- heart rate, CHF—chronic heart failure, LV EF—left ventricular ejection fraction, ECG—electrocardiogram, MET—Metabolic equivalent, used for the assessment of baseline physical activity and exercise tolerance during stress tests, measured through the determination of peak oxygen consumption—VO_2 at rest.

Table 1.
Risk stratification (RR) protocols for CVD patients participating in cardiac rehabilitation (CR).

in turn, leads to the expansion of muscle blood circulation, increasing venous return and cardiac output [11]. In physical training, the proportional contribution of the change in heart rate to the increase in cardiac output is undoubtedly higher than the proportional contribution of stroke volume. The stroke volume normally reaches its maximum by the time the cardiac output increases only to half of its maximum. Any additional increase in cardiac output is possible only through an increase in the heart rate. The power of the load performed by patients depends not only on central hemodynamics, but also on the processes that develop in the myocardium of the right and left ventricles in chronic heart failure.

The interest of most researchers, including our interest, is focused on assessing the impact of physical training on the functional ability of the cardiovascular system and the physical performance of cardiac surgery patients who have undergone heart surgery.

To assess the condition of patients who have undergone coronary artery bypass grafting (CABG) surgery and the choice of the optimal training program, the analysis of the risk of adverse events associated with physical training, as well as cardiorespiratory readiness, is of ongoing interest. The introduction of strategically new algorithms for preparing cardiac surgery patients for physical training programs of varying intensity, with the transition from constant moderate-intensity training to high-intensity interval training, makes it possible to fundamentally change medical approaches to cardiac rehabilitation after open-heart surgery.

Till now are published 7 international protocols for cardiac risk stratification to conduct effective and safe training programs in adult patients with cardiac pathology, mainly with coronary heart disease. These are the protocols of the American Association for Cardiovascular and Pulmonary Rehabilitation [12], the protocol of the American College of Sports Medicine [13], the American Heart Association [14], the protocol of Frederick Pashkov [15], the protocols of the Brazilian Society Cardiology [16], the French Society of Cardiology [17] and the Spanish Society of Cardiology [18]. An analysis of these protocols showed the lack of uniform standards and discrepancy in this matter [19] (**Table 1**). Differences were valued in the statistical significance range of 5% and in most protocols additional studies were conducted to identify cardiac risk of cardiovascular events. The most used test for these purposes was the ergospirometry test. This method has high specificity and reliability, allows to detect myocardial ischemia, arrhythmias, and most importantly, gives the value of the MET (metabolic equivalent) indicator.

In the Russian clinical guidelines for cardiac rehabilitation and secondary prevention of patients after CABG, there is no risk stratification protocol for the selection of patients after CABG to conduct effective aerobic cardiorespiratory trainings (CRT), only a gradation by functional classes of chronic heart failure (CHF) is presented [20].

With all the above in mind, the aim of our study was to develop new approaches to the selection of patients after CABG for the efficient and safe aerobic CRT.

2. Materials and methods

2.1 Study design and study subjects

The study included 137 patients (70 men, 67 women, mean age 68.5 ± 8.3 years) after CABG at the A.N. Bakulev National Medical Research Center for Cardiovascular

Surgery. 90.4% of patients after CABG were classified as being in first functional class chronic heart failure. Mean left ventricular ejection fraction was 58% ± 5.6. 47.8% of patients underwent on-pump CABG and 52.2% of patients underwent off-pump CABG. In most cases 3 vessel CABG was performed.

After surgery, all patients underwent a set of clinical, instrumental and laboratory research investigations, including standard electrocardiography, a test with physical activity on a treadmill/ergospirometry test, a 6-minute walk test, Holter ECG monitoring, transthoracic echocardiography, as well as standard laboratory examinations: complete blood count (hemoglobin, erythrocytes, hematocrit, platelets, leukocytes), biochemical blood test (total protein, albumin, creatinine, urea, alanine aminotransferase - ALT, aspartate aminotransferase - AST, glucose, potassium, sodium, total cholesterol, low and high density lipoproteins) and blood coagulation status (prothrombin time, international normalized ratio, activated partial thromboplastin time, degree of platelet aggregation).

Prior to surgery, all patients underwent coronary angiography, duplex scanning of the extracranial part of the brachiocephalic arteries and arteries of the lower extremities.

Patients who were unable to perform a 6-minute walk test, with a hemoglobin level of less than 95 g/l, with an ALT level of more than 40 U/l, hepatitis, liver dysfunction, liver cirrhosis, and with Gilbert's disease were excluded from the study. Patients with neurological disorders were also excluded from the study. Orthopedic disorders and severe atherosclerosis of the arteries of the lower extremities, which limited the ability to participate in training programs were also among exclusion criteria. The clinical characteristics of patients are presented in **Table 2**.

Major endpoints of the study included: risk stratification of adverse events associated with exercise training after CABG, determination of groups of patients with low, medium, and high levels of physical readiness for aerobic physical CRT of different intensity based on the use of clinical, instrumental and laboratory indicators such as the FIT-treadmill index, ALT (alanine aminotransferase) and the level of postoperative hemoglobin. Study design is presented as **Figure 2**.

Variables	Patients after CABG
Number of patients, n, absolute number	137
On pump CABG/ off pump CABG (%)	47.8%/52.2%
Male	51%
Female	49%
Mean age (years)	68.5 ± 8.3
Body mass index	26.8 ± 5
METs	6.3 ± 0.3
Mean left ventricular ejection fraction (%)	58 ± 5.6
Chronic heart failure class I (number of patients %)	100%

MET—Metabolic equivalent is the amount of exertion that corresponds to a state of rest. MET is measured through the determination of peak oxygen consumption—VO_2 at rest. It represents the baseline physical activity level.

Table 2.
Clinical characteristics of patients assigned to cardiorespiratory trainings (CRT).

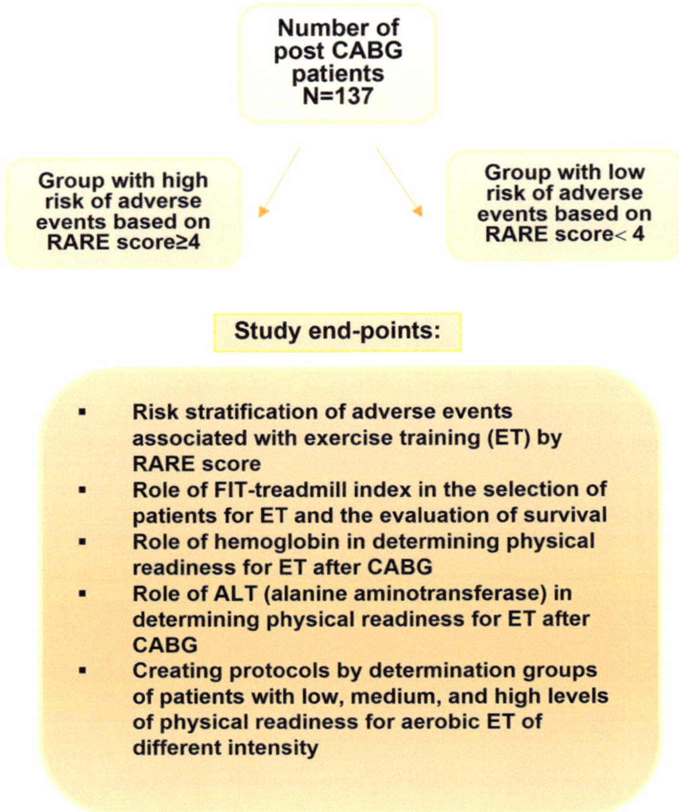

Figure 2.
Study design.

2.2 Exercise protocol

For exercise training in our study, we used ERG 911 bicycle ergometers manufactured by Schiller (Switzerland). Aerobic physical training on bicycle ergometers was carried out for 4 weeks: it started 30 days after the surgery and then continued on an outpatient basis. In the first 7 days, training was carried out with a *Pulse-steady-state protocol*, the second week - with *a ramp interval protocol*. First week the duration of the exercises was on average 20 minutes, in the second week – 30–35 minutes.

In a *pulse-steady-state protocol*, heart rate training and ergometer load are interrelated, with the ergometer load being an adjustable parameter. The load of the ergometer is adjusted to maintain a constant “training heart rate”. In addition to the training itself, this program is very suitable as a reference for comparing with other training programs. The exercise regimen was calculated using ergospirometry data based on the maximal or peak VO_2.

The *ramp interval protocol* is a protocol with a linear increase in load between two levels with heart rate control. The workload in this program includes two levels, which replace each other. The load at which the training heart rate is first reached serves as a reference load to determine the lower return point, calculated by subtracting a certain value from the upper load level. As soon as the training heart rate is reached the load will be continuously reduced to the lowest point of return.

Regarding the intensity of aerobic physical training, we used trainings of moderate and high intensity. In moderate intensity training the goal was to reach 60–75% of peak oxygen consumption (VO_2). In high-intensity training, the goal was to reach 80–85% of peak oxygen consumption (VO_2). The choice of training intensity method was based on the patients' belonging to certain groups and a linear relationship between heart rate and VO_2. In our study we used high-intensity interval training (HIIT) programs with a 4-minute high-intensity workout regimen followed by intermediate 3-minute rest breaks (Nordic model) as well as constant training programs of moderate intensity (MICT). The intensity and mode of training were determined individually depending on the level of physical readiness of patients based on the developed algorithm. As a follow up, patients were advised to continue physical training individually based on the selected type of training. Remote monitoring of exercising patients within the study lasted from 4 months (120 days) to 1 year to assess survival, mortality, and morbidity.

2.3 Assessment of risks associated with physical training

One of the main endpoints of our study was to determine the predictive role of the RARE scale in the development of adverse events due to physical training on the example of our patients after CABG.

Patients were divided into groups depending on the low or high risk of adverse events according to the well-known and generally accepted scale of assessment of risks associated with physical training (RARE score) [21]. The RARE (risk of activity related event) scale considers resting heart rate, resting blood pressure, functional activity in METs, ischemic events according to the well-known classification of angina pectoris and ST segment changes, left ventricular ejection fraction, and the presence or absence of arrhythmias. Each of the indicators is assigned a value from 0 to 4, except for heart rate and blood pressure, which are assigned 2 points. The RARE scale is determined by summing the scores of all six of the above indicators and can range from 0 to 20 points. Patients with a score of ≥4 are at high risk of adverse events, and patients with a score of <4 are at low risk.

In the RARE scale, there are 5 large criteria, which are assigned 4 points: <6.0 METS exercise tolerance, LVEF <20% (left ventricular ejection fraction), recurrent VT (ventricular tachycardia)/VF(ventricular fibrillation) in the absence of AMI (acute myocardial infarction), or severe ischemia (III-IV FC according to the Canadian classification CCS, ST-segment depression more than 2 mm, multivessel lesion of the coronary arteries/proximal significant stenosis of anterior interventricular descendance or stenosis of the trunk of the left coronary artery. Thus, the RARE score identifies high-risk patients with a combination of small criteria, such as hypotension with moderate left ventricular dysfunction, atrial fibrillation (AFIB) with a frequent ventricular response, or angina pectoris II FC according to CCS with a moderate decrease in exercise tolerance.

The group of higher risk of developing adverse events during physical training on the RARE scale included patients of the older age group, female, with diabetes and hypertension, and a high body mass index (**Table 3**). Carotid atherosclerosis was prevalent in the higher risk group.

2.4 Assessment of survival by FIT treadmill index

There are 3 components to physical training: frequency (how many times a week the training takes place), intensity (how intense the load is during training), and time

Variables	Low risk (n = 96)	High risk (n = 41)	p
Age, years	61 ± 11	67 ± 10	<0.001
Gender m/f, (number of patients %)	M-77%/F-23%	M- 48%/F- 52%	0.017
Waist, size in cm	85 ± 13	108 ± 16	<0.001
Weight, kg	86.8 ± 17.5	88.5 ± 21.4	0.3
Body mass index kg/m^2	29.6 ± 5.3	31.1 ± 6.9	0.03
Heart rate, beat/min	67 ± 13	67 ± 14	0.483
SAP, mmHg	118 ± 15	121 ± 19	0.02
DAP, mmHg	73 ± 9	71 ± 11	0.034
Left ventricular EF, (%)	61.5 ± 8.6	56.5 ± 13.5	<0.001
METs	8.4 ± 1.9	5.8 ± 1.5	<0.001
Total cholesterol, mmol/l	3.56 ± 1.01	3.7 ± 1.2	0.087
HDLP mmol/l	1.17 ± 0.31	1.15 ± 0.34	0.481
LDLP mmol/l	1.8 ± 0.82	1.88 ± 0.95	0.26
TG, mmol/l	1.3 ± 0.77	1.53 ± 1.39	0.007
HbA_{1c},%	6.1 ± 0.8	6.7 ± 1.2	<0.001
Arterial hypertension (%)	49	60	0.004
Diabetes type 2 (%)	21	36	<0.001
AT of carotid arteries, %	8	20	0.002

Table 3.
Characteristics of post CABG patients with low risk (< 4 points) or high risk (≥4 points) of developing adverse events associated with physical trainings based on RARE score.

(how long the training lasts). All these 3 points make up the FIT formula (F = frequency, I = intensity, T = time). By correctly combining all 3 points trainings can be planned most effectively.

With the advent of fitness, it became possible to establish a reliable survival rate in patients engaged in fitness, that is, aerobic cardiorespiratory and other types of training. As part of Henry Ford's Physical Training Testing and Evaluation Project, the FIT treadmill score (FIT treadmill index) was calculated [22]. It allows clinicians to calculate and predict the 10-year risk of survival and mortality in healthy individuals and fitness patients.

FIT treadmill index =85% maximal predictive HR + 12 × (METs)-4 × (age) +43 if the patient is female.

Survival = 0.014 (%Max. predictive heart rate + 0.182 (METs) + 0.6381 (female) - 0.0613 (age).

FIT treadmill index was adjusted after CRT (cardiorespiratory training) programs: FIT treadmill index ≥100 meant very low mortality risk, FIT treadmill index 1–100 defined low risk, ≤0 to −100 - intermediate risk, ≤ − 100 to −200 high risk. FIT treadmill index ≥100 is associated with 2% risk of mortality in 10 years. FIT treadmill index between "-100" and "-200" is associated with 38% risk of mortality in 10 years.

The Treadmill FIT Index serves as a quantitative expression of cardiorespiratory fitness for participation in training programs. It's easy to calculate. It does not depend on symptoms, and is not limited to electrocardiographic changes, but includes age factor and gender in the calculation of risk. Moreover, in addition to determining the risk during training programs and prognosis of coronary artery stenosis, it makes it possible to predict long-term survival. The METs indicator is decisive and universal in the selection of patients for cardiac rehabilitation, and the FIT index, in the calculation of which METs is used, can serve as an additional factor for determining cardiorespiratory fitness.

2.5 Blood measurements

All patients underwent a complete blood count with the determination of hemoglobin, erythrocytes, platelets, leukocytes; biochemical blood test, including AST, ALT, glucose, creatinine, alkaline phosphatase, lipid profile. ALT activity was assessed using the standard Beckman Coulter test. Quantification was carried out using kinetic UV tests. In order to ensure the maximum catalytic activity of the ALT level in the blood, activated peroxidase phosphate, which is a necessary co-factor for the catalytic activity of ALT, was added to all tubes.

In our center, the following reference values have been determined: ALT 10–40 U/L, AST 10–42 U/L.

The reference values of the lipid profile are as follows: total cholesterol 3.1–5.2 mmol/L, Triglycerides 0.4–1.81 mmol/L, HDL 0.75–2.31 mmol/L, LDL 0–3.9 mmol/L, creatinine 53–115 μmol/L.

2.6 Statistical analysis

Statistical data processing was carried out using SPSS 22.0 and SAS, version 9.3. The indicators are represented by mean and standard deviation (M ± SD) data. Qualitative indicators were presented in % of the total number of patients in the sample or in the corresponding group. To compare the performance of the two groups, the chi-square test, the Fisher (F) test for small samples, the Wilcoxon Matched Pairs Test, the Mann-Whitney U Test, and its modification of the Mann and Whitney U-test were used. In the case of more than two independent samples (in the analysis of indicators in 3 groups), the H-test according to the Kruskal method and Wallis (Kruskal - Wallis one-way analysis of variance) was used. In the case of a near-normal distribution, the Student's test was also used to compare the two samples. Correlation analysis was performed using Spearman's rank correlation. The differences were considered statistically significant at $p < 0.05$.

A univariate regression analysis was performed using Fisher's x2 test and Student's t-test. Statistically significant parameters ($p < 0.05$) were introduced into a multivariate regression analysis (generalized logistic model) to identify independent predictors; The selection of significant features was carried out using a standard step-by-step procedure with the inclusion of variables. Survival curves were assessed using the Kaplan-Meier method and a hazard ratio with a 95% confidence interval.

3. Results

3.1 The risk stratification of adverse events associated with physical trainings after CABG

A total of 11 adverse events were recorded in the study, including 8 events in the high-risk group and 3 events in the low-risk group. All these were small events

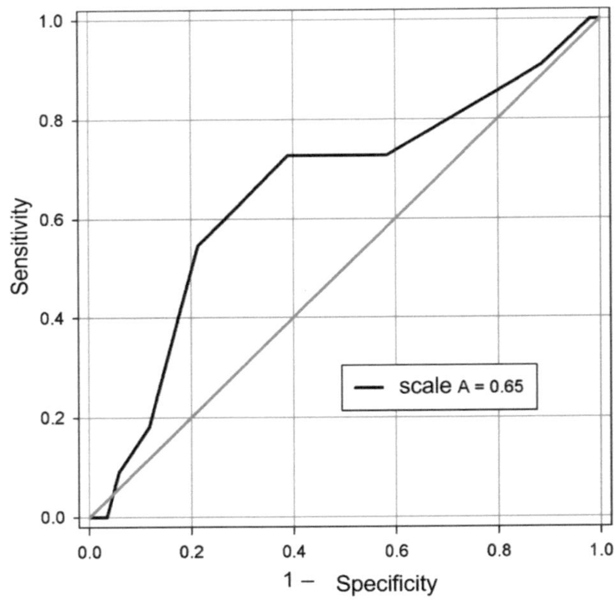

Figure 3.
The dependence of the sensitivity of the RARE scale on the frequency of false-positive conclusions (p = 0.024).

– symptomatic hypotension, hypertension, symptomatic tachycardia, in one case a short episode of atrial fibrillation (AF), ventricular bigeminy and ST-depression up to 1 mm along the anterolateral wall of the LV. The development of adverse events in our study associated with aerobic CRT is low 0.8% (11 adverse events per 1370 hours of training).

Analysis of the dependence of the sensitivity of the scale on the frequency of false-positive results showed the diagnostic reliability of the threshold value of the RARE scale ≥4 points in assessing the risk of developing adverse events due to physical training. According to linear regression analysis high-risk group had a significant predictive significance in the development of low-risk events (R = 0.09, B = 0.023, P = 0,024) and there was a tendency to increase the risk of adverse events with the growth in the RARE scale (relative risk 4.2; X^2 = 5,12; p = 0.024, power 0.62) (**Figure 3**).

The low positive predictive value of the RARE score of 3.1% according to linear regression analysis in our study indicates that it is necessary to concentrate on identifying patients who have a low, rather than high, risk of developing adverse events during physical training. In this respect, the RARE scale accurately gives the possibility to determine patients with low risk, since none of the patients in this group had large/significant complications and the vast majority were free from any events in the long-term period.

3.2 The role of laboratory parameters in the selection of patients after CABG for aerobic CRT

When determining the role of laboratory parameters for the selection of groups after CABG with a low, medium, and high level of readiness for aerobic CRT, attention was focused on 2 indicators of hemoglobin and ALT levels. According to the recommendations of the European Society of Cardiothoracic Surgeons, the hemoglobin level ≤ 100 g/l after CABG is considered the threshold for entry into cardiac rehabilitation programs and it is proposed to refrain from starting aerobic CRT [23]. With hemoglobin of 100 g/l or less, the tolerance to physical activity, determined by the test with a 6-minute walk, is significantly lower.

In our study, a hemoglobin level of 100 g/L was detected in 55 (40.15%) out of 137 patients (including 10 women, 45 men) before the onset of CRT. In 82 patients (60%), the hemoglobin value was more than 100 g/l and ranged from 100 to 130 g/l. Before the onset of aerobic CRT in the subgroup of patients with hemoglobin 95–100 g/l, the average distance during the 6-minute walk test was 258 ± 106 meters, while in the subgroup of patients with hemoglobin more than 100 g/l 306 ± 101 meters (p = 0.007). The maximum METs on the treadmill, the maximum heart rate and the threshold heart rate were significantly lower in the hemoglobin group of 95–100 g/L. Depression of the ST segment of a non-ischemic nature, as well as the inversion of the T-wave and single VE during exercise also occurred significantly more often in patients with hemoglobin 95–100 g/l. At a hemoglobin level of 100 g/l or less, the distance covered in meters during a 6-minute walk test was significantly lower, and in these patients, there was a significant increase in that distance after the course of CRT.

Generally, in all patients, the average distance in meters for 6 minutes increased from 298 ± 100 meters (before the onset of CRT) to 431 ± 90 meters at the end of the CRT course (p = 0.001) (**Table 4**). Thus, even if exercise tolerance is reduced with a hemoglobin value of less than 100 g/l, the absolute value of the 6-minute walk test is acceptable (200 m). Moreover, this "gap" in exercise tolerance is fully restored in 7 weeks (49 days) of CRT, when physical fitness no longer depends on hemoglobin values.

It has been proven and known that the alanine aminotransferase - ALT threshold level of ≤17 U/L is associated with an increased probability of long-term mortality in patients with coronary heart disease [24, 25]. Considering the significant prognostic role of ALT in large studies, we divided our patients into groups depending on the ALT serum level.

It turned out that in the group of patients with an ALT level of ≤17 U/L, exercise tolerance measured in METs and exercise duration was significantly lower, resting heart rate was significantly higher and reserve heart rate was significantly lower (**Table 5**).

In addition, the level of ALT ≤17 U/L was most significantly associated with (p 0.001) older age (≥67 years), body mass index (≤25.8) and female gender. When

Hemoglobin (g/l)	Distance in meters by 6 min walk test before CRT	p (between groups)	Distance in meters by 6 min walk test after CRT	p(between groups)
95–100	258 ± 106		415 ± 73	
100–130	306 ± 101	0.007	437 ± 95	0.166

Table 4.
Distance covered by 6-minute walk test in patients with different hemoglobin level before and after cardiac respiratory trainings (CRT).

	ALT≤17 U/l	ALT≤40 U/l	
METs	6.86 ± 0.2	7.83 ± 1.5	p 0.01
Test duration (min, sec)	6 min 41 sec ± 1.5 min	8 min 44 sec ± 2.5 min	p 0.01
Rest heart rate, beat/min	72 ± 13	65 ± 10	p 0.01
Reserve heart rate beat/min	49 ± 24	54 ± 24	p 0.01
Max. Systolic AP mmHg	164 ± 34	161 ± 27	p 0.44

Table 5.
Comparative analysis of MOD-Bruce treadmill stress-tests based on ALT level.

included in a multivariate regression analysis, hemoglobin≤100 g/L and ALT≤17 U/L independently of each other, and from other indicators, were associated with reduced exercise tolerance and thus with reduced cardiorespiratory suitability for cardiorespiratory training after CABG.

3.3 The role of the FIT treadmill index in the determination of cardiorespiratory fitness and the prediction of survival after CABG

In our study, 137 patients after CABG were followed up for 1 year. Before entering the cardiac rehabilitation program with the use of aerobic CRT, the average level of METs according to the BRUCE protocol was 6.3 ± 0.3. In 4-weeks of aerobic CRT, the average level of METs according to the BRUCE protocol was 8.3 ± 2.2 and exercise tolerance significantly increased by an average of 2.0 ± 1.2 METs. ($p \leq 0.05$).

By risk category, before the start of aerobic CRT, 70% of our patients had a low probable risk of mortality (respectively, a high estimated survival rate) and 30% of patients had an intermediate probable risk of mortality according to the FIT-treadmill index. Considering the average age of our patients 68.5 to 8.3 years and an almost equal proportion of men and women (70 men, 67 women), the initial average of the FIT treadmill index was −69-59.5. After a 4-week course of aerobic CRT, the average FIT treadmill index was "-30.963.3". Thus, the average improvement in the FIT treadmill index was 38,110.2 points. ($p \leq 0.05$).

30% of patients who had an initially probable intermediate risk of mortality according to the FIT treadmill index (they also had a relatively high risk of adverse events based on the RARE scale>4), after a 4-week course of aerobic CRT using constant moderate intensity exercises, moved to the group with a low probable risk of mortality.

In a comparative analysis of the sensitivity, specificity, and predictive reliability of METs, the percentage of the maximum predictive heart rate (%Max. predictive HR) and the FIT-Treadmill index, the FIT-Treadmill index was statistically the most reliable (**Figure 4**). When analyzing the degree of improvement of the FIT-treadmill index after aerobic CRT, we identified a threshold value for an increase in FIT-Treadmill index score of 18.2 points with specificity of 76% (CI = confidence interval 68.1%–80.49%) and sensitivity of 68% (CI 52.9%–79.7%). Estimated survival rates were shown at 1 year.

Thus, the FIT treadmill index provides a quantitative measurement of cardiorespiratory fitness and allows to predict long-term survival. Obviously, participation in the cardiac rehabilitation program significantly improves the FIT-treadmill index.

DOI: http://dx.doi.org/10.5772/intechopen.1003996

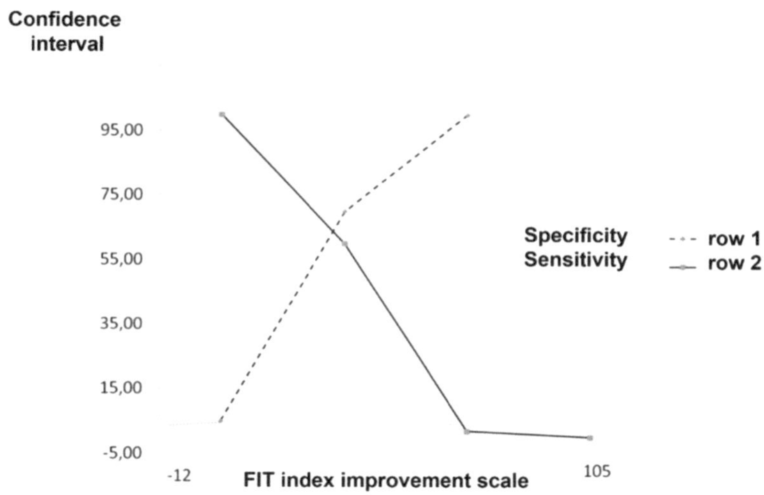

Figure 4.
FIT treadmill index sensitivity and specificity in post CABG survival prediction.

3.4 Developed algorithms for the selection and risk stratification of patients for the efficient cardiorespiratory trainings after CABG

Conducted univariate and then multivariate regression analysis resulted in an algorithm for assessing the readiness and the risk of participation in aerobic CRT programs for patients after CABG.

Algorithm for the high level of readiness for aerobic CRT and for the low risk of adverse events after CABG in the presence of one of the following or more criteria determined the following variables:

- Uncomplicated postoperative course
- Exercise tolerance ≥7 METs
- < 4 points by RARE score.
- Absence of myocardial ischemia
- LV EF >50%
- Absence of high-grade ventricular arrhythmias according to Lown classification
- The level of the FIT treadmill index 1–100
- Blood ALT level ≥ 17 U/l
- The level of hemoglobin in the blood ≥100 g/l

Algorithm for the low level of readiness for aerobic CRT and an average risk of adverse events after CABG in the presence of one of the following or more criteria determined the following variables:

- The presence of angina pectoris
- Reversible deviations based on the results of a stress test on a treadmill
- Exercise tolerance 6–7 METs
- $\leq$ 4 points by RARE score.
- EF LV 45–50%
- FIT-treadmill Index level from −56,9 до −30,9 ($\leq$0 to −100)
- Blood ALT level $\leq$ 17 U/l
- The level of hemoglobin in the blood $\leq$100 g/l

4. Discussion

It has been found that in trained people, regardless of their risk factor profile, mortality from cardiovascular events over a 30-year period is 50% lower than in untrained or poorly trained, i.e. physically inactive people [26]. Compared to less physically active men, the risk of cardiovascular events was shown to decrease progressively with increasing levels of cardiorespiratory fitness, especially among individuals with high and very high Agatson calcium index scores [27].

Patients who have undergone CABG have several limiting physical activity features such as deterioration of the function of external respiration with a decrease in respiratory volume, pain syndrome with little physical exertion, during breathing, decreased muscle strength due to immobilization. The presence of following "syndrome complexes" should be taken into account in the formation of physical rehabilitation measures: cardiac, post-sternotomy, respiratory, hemorheological, psychopathological, hemodynamic, metabolic and post-phlebectomy. This population of patients is recommended mobilization, including both active and breathing passive exercises. In the case of positive dynamics in the postoperative period, it is advisable to start with physical aerobic cardiorespiratory training. Cardiac rehabilitation including exercise training is indicated for all patients after CABG [28]. Our previous studies have shown positive effects of aerobic exercise training on metabolic and cardiorespiratory response in study group after CABG compared to control group without any training programs involved [29]. These positive effects were more obvious in high-intensity training group compared to moderate-intensity continuous training group [$p < 0.01$] in 4 weeks of trainings after CABG. Systematic physical training 3 times a week for 4–6 months in patients who have undergone CABG was associated with a significant increase in tolerance to physical activity up to 50% by 12 months and peak oxygen consumption, decrease of elevated heart rate (HR), improved daily physical activity and cholesterol concentration, level of high-density lipoproteins and improved quality of life.

Before embarking on a particular program of physical cardiac rehabilitation, a thorough assessment of the clinical and functional status of the patient is necessary, which should make it possible to create a risk stratification protocol: calculate the level of physical readiness for choosing the intensity of physical training, further planning a rehabilitation program; to assess the possible risks of various adverse events, cardiovascular morbidity and mortality in the long-term period after such operations.

Comparative analysis of 7 international protocols for cardiac risk stratification to conduct effective and safe training programs in adult patients with coronary artery disease did not allow to determine the best protocol for stratifying the risk of participation in training programs [19]. The analysis showed that none of these protocols was effective in such a prognosis and did not allow patients to be classified as at high risk of developing complications due to low positive predictive significance and low sensitivity (**Table 1**). The predictive significance of the protocols was greatest when used in the combination. It has been suggested that such encouraging results were due to a combination of the absence of potential risk predictors and the low incidence of serious complications during training programs. Although several protocols suggested using the risk stratification criteria associated with increased morbidity and mortality in the general population, it remained unclear whether the overall risk of cardiac events and the risk during training programs were the same phenomenon. Stratification criteria included factors associated with an increased risk of morbidity and mortality during physical training. However, the existence of multitude single-center protocols made it difficult to standardize the approach to the correct selection of patients for effective CRT programs.

When stratifying the risk of various complications, it is advisable and most effective to use both cardiac risk factors, as well as the assessment of non-cardiac comorbidities such as diabetes mellitus, chronic obstructive pulmonary disease, cerebrovascular disease, and peripheral arterial disease.

The purpose of our research was to create a new algorithm for the selection of patients after CABG for effective and safe aerobic cardiorespiratory training. The results of aerobic cardiorespiratory training, as well as survival and morbidity, were evaluated within a year after surgery.

To determine the risk of adverse events associated with physical training, the international RARE scale was used, which considers heart rate, resting blood pressure, functional activity in METs, ischemic events according to the well-known classification of angina pectoris and ST-segment changes, left ventricular ejection fraction, and the presence or absence of arrhythmias.

The risk of adverse events associated with physical training in the study was extremely low, 0.8%, which is consistent with the data of other investigators. A high diagnostic reliability of the threshold value of the RARE scale ≥4 points in assessing the risk of developing adverse events due to physical training was shown.

The obtained protocol to determine the level of readiness to perform aerobic CRT after CABG included the following parameters: exercise tolerance in METs, RARE scale, FIT treadmill index, left ventricular ejection fraction, hemoglobin, and ALT levels.

The hemoglobin level ≤ 100 g/l did not serve as an obstacle to the onset of aerobic CRT, since it determined a reliably acceptable tolerance to physical activity on a 6-minute walk test and proved a significant restoration of the gap in cardiorespiratory capacity after a course of physical training.

The FIT-treadmill index was used to calculate long-term survival, as it is the powerful predictor of mortality with predictive power independent of age, gender, left ventricular ejection fraction and other traditional cardiovascular risk factors. It is easy to calculate. It is independent of symptoms and is not limited to electrocardiographic changes.

International risk stratification protocols for the selection of patients for the purpose of safe and effective CRT include neither the RARE scale, nor the FIT-treadmill Index, or laboratory parameters. Thus, a distinctive feature of our protocol is the ability to assess the logical pattern of the relationship of certain indicators with cardiorespiratory fitness and the possible risk of adverse events due to CRT, as well as the likelihood of assessing long-term survival in actively exercising and non-exercising patients. Groups of patients after CABG with low and high levels of readiness for physical cardiac rehabilitation were defined. It is necessary for the safe and effective performance of moderate- or high-intensity aerobic CRT in continuous or interval regimens.

Increasing the number of cardiac patients with concomitant pathology imposes the search and development of new criteria for efficient and safe cardiac rehabilitation after open heart surgery. The growing interest in this problem justifies the increase in the number of training programs offered. The proposed protocol for the management of patients after CABG contains a multiplicity of specific terms for

	High intensity interval trainings (HIIT)			**p**		
Variables	**0 weeks**	**2 weeks**	**4 weeks**	**Inside group**	**Comparison between HIIT and MICT (p)**	
VO_2(ml/kg/min)	23.5 ± 5.7	26.7 ± 5.7	30.6 ± 6.9	$***_{a,b,c}$	*	Significant
HR (beat/min)	134 ± 21	140 ± 19	147 ± 18.2	$***_{a,b,c}$	**	Significant
Power load (Wt)	154 ± 38.8	177 ± 45	192 ± 46.9	$***_{a,b,c}$	*	Significant
RER	1.26 ± 0.12	1.27 ± 0.12	1.28 ± 0.11	NS	NS	NS
O_2 pulse ml/beat/min	14.8 ± 3.6	16 ± 3.5	18.6 ± 3.5	$***_{a,b,c}$	NS	NS
	Moderate intensity continuous trainings (MICT)					
VO_2(ml/kg/min)	22.4 ± 5.6	25.2 ± 6.2	27.8 ± 6.7	$***_{a,b,c}$	*	Significant
HR (beat/min)	129 ± 21.1	133 ± 22.3	138 ± 21.5	$***_{a,b,c}$	**	Significant
Power load (Wt)	145 ± 41	169 ± 47.9	180 ± 46.6	$***_{a,b,c}$	*	Significant
RER	1.26 ± 0.11	1.26 ± 0.09	1.27 ± 0.09	NS	NS	NS
O_2 pulse ml/beat/min	14.7 ± 2.9	15.9 ± 3.3	16.7 ± 3.2	$***_{a,b}$	NS	NS

[a] *variables in 2 weeks significantly differed from baseline.*
[b] *variables in 4 weeks significantly differed from baseline.*
[c] *variables in 4 weeks significantly differed from variables in 2 weeks of CRT.*
**$p < 0.05$; **$p < 0.01$; ***$p < 0.001$; NS—nonsignificant, HR—heart rate.*
O_2-pulse—it is the volume of O_2 that the blood absorbs with each contraction of the heart. O_2-pulse = (VO_2/HR). Normal values: 11–17 ml/beat/min.
RER respiratory exchange ratio—this is the ratio of O_2 consumed and CO_2 products. The RER reflects the level of transition from the aerobic supply zone to the anaerobic zone. At the time of transition from aerobic to anaerobic mode, the respiratory coefficient becomes equal to 1. The maximum value of the RER > 1 characterizes the maximum speed endurance.

Table 6.
Comparative analysis of VO2, heart rate, power load, RER and O2 pulse.

monitoring the effectiveness of the measures taken, predictors by which the quality and efficiency of each individual case can be assessed.

Clinical implementation of our algorithms resulted in positive effects on metabolism, physiology, and hemodynamics of cardiovascular system. 96 patients with a high level of readiness for aerobic CRT and a low risk of adverse events were offered a transition from aerobic cardiorespiratory training of moderate intensity for 2 days to high-intensity interval aerobic cardiorespiratory training (HIIT). 41 patients with a low level of readiness for physical training and an average risk of adverse events were offered only moderate intensity continuous training (MICT). Aerobic cardiorespiratory trainings were carried out for 4 weeks under clinical observation.

In our study moderate intensity aerobic CRT was defined as a training when 60–75% of peak oxygen consumption or 60–75% of maximum training heart rate was achieved, and high-intensity aerobic CRT was defined as a training in which 80–85% of peak oxygen consumption or 80–85% of the maximum training heart rate was achieved.

As a result of aerobic CRTs, the indicators of peak oxygen consumption significantly improved - VO_2 (peak oxygen consumption), HR, power load and oxygen pulse ($p < 0,001$). VO_2, HR and power load significantly increased more in the HIIT group than in the MICT group (**Table 6**). In both groups, after aerobic CRT of high and medium intensity, there was a significant decrease in weight, body mass index (BMI), resting heart rate, a decrease in systolic and diastolic blood pressure, to a greater extent diastolic blood pressure, and an improvement in high-density lipoproteins (HDL) and a significant decrease in triglyceride levels, but the atherogenic coefficient did not change. From the baseline echocardiography parameters for the 4-week period of aerobic CRT, we observed a statistically significant decrease in the end-diastolic volume of the left ventricle (p 0.025) and an increase in LVEF (0.003), to a greater extent in the HIIT group. *These observations confirm the positive effects of aerobic cardiorespiratory training on the physiology and hemodynamics of the cardiovascular system, lipid and carbohydrate metabolism.*

The created algorithm for selecting patients allows safe and efficient usage of aerobic training programs of moderate and high intensity in continuous or interval modes, depending on the level of risk and the patient's cardiorespiratory readiness. All this ensures the earliest possible start of cardiac rehabilitation programs, their continuity and duration.

Author details

Tea Kakuchaya*, Leo Bockeria, Zarina Tokaeva, Nona Pachuashvili and Tamara Dzhitava
AN Bakulev National Medical Research Center of Cardiovascular Surgery, Moscow, Russia

*Address all correspondence to: kakuchinit@yahoo.com; ttkakuchaya@gmail.com

References

[1] Paul Wood's Diseases of the Heart and Circulation. Eyre & Spottiswoode in English. 3rd ed. Lippincott, University of California; 1968. p. 1164. Open Library OL5639268M, LCCN 68068633

[2] Ponikowski et al. 2016 ESC guidelines for the diagnosis and treatment of acute and chronic heart failure: The task force for the diagnosis and treatment of acute and chronic heart failure of the European Society of Cardiology (ESC)Developed with the special contribution of the Heart Failure Association (HFA) of the ESC. European Heart Journal. 14 Jul 2016;**37**(27):2129-2200

[3] Rauch B, Davos CH, Doherty P, et al. The prognostic effect of cardiac rehabilitation in the era of acute revascularisation and statin therapy: A systematic review and meta-analysis of randomized and non-randomized studies – The cardiac rehabilitation outcome study (CROS). European Journal of Preventive Cardiology. 2016;**23**(18):1914-1939. DOI: 10.1177/2047487316671181

[4] Anderson L, Oldridge N, Thompson DR, et al. Exercise-based cardiac rehabilitation for coronary heart disease. Journal of the American College of Cardiology. 2016;**67**(1):1-12. DOI: 10.1016/j.jacc.2015.10.044

[5] Wang J-S. Exercise prescription and thrombogenesis. Journal of Biomedical Science. 2006;**13**:753-761. DOI: 10.1007/s11373-006-9105-7

[6] Kachur S, Chongthammakun V, Lavie CJ, et al. Impact of cardiac rehabilitation and exercise training programs in coronary heart disease. Progress in Cardiovascular Diseases. 2017;**60**:103-114. DOI: 10.1016/j.pcad.2017.07.002

[7] Soci UPR, Fernandes T, Barauna VG, et al. Epigenetic control of exercise training-induced cardiac hypertrophy by miR-208. Clinical Science (London). 1 Nov 2016;**130**(22):2005-2015. DOI: 10.1042/CS20160480

[8] Krzeminski K. The role of adrenomedullin in cardiovascular response to exercise - a review. Journal of Human Kinetics. 2016;**53**:127-142. DOI: 10.1515/hukin-2016-0017

[9] Smart NA, Meyer T, Butterfield JA, et al. Individual patient meta-analysis of exercise training effects on systemic brain natriuretic peptide expression in heart failure. European Journal of Preventive Cardiology. 2012;**19**(3):428-435. DOI: 10.1177/1741826711409171

[10] Barcroft H, Dornhors AC. Blood flow through human calf during rhythmic exercise. The Journal of Physiology. 1949;**109**:402

[11] Guyton AC, Jones CE, Coleman TB. Circulatory Physiology: Cardiac Output and ITS Regulation. Philadelphia: WB Saunders Co; 1973

[12] American Association of Cardiovascular and Pulmonary Rehabilitation. Diretrizes Para reabilitação cardíaca e Programas de prevenção secundária Marx AG, Translator. 4th ed. São Paulo: Roca; 2007. p. 244

[13] American College of Sports Medicine. Diretrizes Do ACSM Para o Teste de esforço e Sua prescrição. Taranto G, translator. 7th ed. Rio de Janeiro: Guanabara Koogan; 2007. 239

[14] Fletcher GF, Balady GJ, Amsterdam EA, Chaitman B, Eckel R,

Fleg J, et al. Exercise standards for testing and training: A statement for healthcare professionals from the American Heart Association. Circulation. 2001;**104**(14):1694-1740. DOI: 10.1161/hc3901.095960

[15] Pashkow FJ. Issues in contemporary cardiac rehabilitation: A historical perspective. Journal of the American College of Cardiology. 1993;**21**(3):822-834. DOI: 10.1016/0735-1097(93)90116-I

[16] Moraes RS. Diretriz de Reabilitação Cardíaca. Arquivos Brasileiros de Cardiologia. 2005;**84**(5):431-440

[17] Monpère C, Sellier P, Meurin P, Aeberhard PB, D'Agrosa Boiteux M, Iliou M, et al. Recommandations de la Société française de cardiologie concernant la pratique de la réadaptation cardiovasculaire chez l'adulte. Version 2. Archives des maladies du coeur et des vaisseaux. 2002;**95**(10):962-997

[18] Velasco JA, Cosín J, Maroto JM, Muñiz J, Casasnovas JA, Plaza I, et al. Guías de práctica clínica de la Sociedad Española de Cardiología en prevencíon cardiovascular y rehabilitación cardíaca. Revista Española de Cardiología. 2000;**53**(8):1095-1120. DOI: 10.1016/S0300-8932(00)75211-0

[19] Santos AAS, Anne KF, Silva1 FM. Vanderlei analysis of agreement between cardiac risk stratification protocols applied to participants of a center for cardiac rehabilitation. Brazilian Journal of Physical Therapy. 2016;**20**(4):298-305

[20] Bockeria LA, Aronov DM. Russian clinical recommendations. Coronary artery bypass grafting in patients with ischemic heart disease. Rehabilitation and Secondary Prevention. Cardiosomatics. 2016;7(№3-№4):5-71

[21] Lacombe SP, LaHaye SA, Hopkins-Rosseel D, Ball D, Lau W. Identifying patients at low risk for activity-related events: The RARE score. Journal of Cardiopulmonary Rehabilitation and Prevention. 2014;**34**(3):180-187

[22] Cuenza LR, Emily Mae LY, Edgardo E. Assessment of the prognostic utility of the FIT treadmill score in coronary artery disease patients undergoing cardiac rehabilitation. Journal of Cardiovascular and Thoracic Research. 2019;**11**(1):8-13. DOI: 10.15171/jcvtr.2019.02 Epub 2019 Feb 5

[23] Ranucci M, La Rovere MT, Castelvecchio S, Maestri R, Menicanti L, Frigiola A, et al. Postoperative anemia and exercise tolerance after cardiac operations in patients without transfusion: What hemoglobin level is acceptable? The Annals of Thoracic Surgery. 2011;**92**(1):25-31

[24] Kogan M, Klempfnerb R, Lotana D, Wasserstruma Y, Goldenbergb I, Segal G. Low ALT blood levels are associated with lower baseline fitness amongst participants of a cardiac rehabilitation program. Journal of Exercise Science and Fitness. 2018;**16**:1-4

[25] Peltz-Sinvani N, Klempfner R, Ramaty E, Sela BA, Goldenberg I, Segal G. Low ALT levels independently associated with 22-year all-cause mortality among coronary heart disease patients. Journal of General Internal Medicine. 2015;**31**(2):209-214

[26] Wickramasinghe CD, Ayers CR, Das S, de Lemos JA, Willis BL, Berry JD. Prediction of 30-year risk for cardiovascular mortality by fitness and risk factor levels: The Cooper Center longitudinal study. Circulation. Cardiovascular Quality and Outcomes. 2014;7:597-602. DOI: 10.1161/CIRCOUTCOMES.113.000531

[27] Radford NB, DeFina LF, Leonard D, Barlow CE, Willis BL, Gibbons LW, et al. Cardiorespiratory fitness, coronary artery calcium, and cardiovascular disease events in a cohort of generally healthy middle-age men: Results from the Cooper Center longitudinal study. Circulation. 2018;**137**:1888-1895. DOI: 10.1161/CIRCULATIONAHA.117.032708

[28] Niebauer J. Is there a role for cardiac rehabilitation after coronary artery bypass grafting? Circulation. 2016;**133**:2529-2537

[29] Kuular A, Kakuchaya T, Dzhitava T, Filatova A, Pachuashvili N. The effect of high-intensity interval physical training on the energy supply system in patients after heart surgery. International Journal of Innovative Medicine. 2022;**2**:4-8. DOI: 10.33667/2782-4101-2022-2-4-8

Chapter 6

Supportive Exercises for Cancer Patients

Hajer Alhinai

Abstract

Cancer is a major health issue that significantly contributes to mortality worldwide. In 2023, an estimated 1,958,310 new cancer cases were projected in the United States. Individuals with cancer may suffer from physical impairments, fatigue, psychological and social issues that reduce their quality of life. Cancer treatments (post-operation, chemotherapy, or radiotherapy) can cause several side effects. Exercises or physical activity are safe and offer a positive impact before, during, and after cancer treatment, encompassing aerobic, resistance, balance, flexibility exercises and others. Exercises improve quality of life, muscle power, and cardiovascular fitness, while also preventing other diseases and reducing the risk of cancer recurrence and death. The aim of this chapter is to clarify exercises' role in cancer patients. The choice of exercises depends on the diagnosis and patient tolerance, considering contraindications. Physical activity programs should be informed by guidelines, and individualized in intensity, duration, type, and frequency to achieve maximum positive impact.

Keywords: oncology, cancer survivors, exercises, physical activity, cancer related symptoms

1. Introduction

Cancer is a major health issue that significantly contributes to mortality worldwide. In 2023, an estimated 1,958,310 new cancer cases and 609,820 cancer deaths were projected in the United States, with over 15.5 million cancer survivors [1]. Cancer survivors may experience long-term health issues that result from the disease, its treatment, and related comorbid conditions. The risk of cancer increases with age. The majority of cancer patients are known to be elderly [2].

Cancer patients require abundant care, especially during the treatment period. Cancer can impact physical, psychological, social, and economic health, leading to dysfunction for many years following treatments, difficulty returning to work, or independent living, and poor quality of life. For example, common side effects of chemotherapy include but are not limited to, neuropathy, fatigue, nausea, bone marrow suppression, and immune system suppression [3]. Radiotherapy side effects may include tightness of skin, loss of range of motion, loss of bone density, secondary pain, fatigue, and whole-body symptoms similar to the effects of chemotherapy [4]. Additionally, possible side effects of surgery may include pain, scar tissue, swelling, and a reduction in mobility and strength in the affected limb [5]. Cancer-related fatigue is one of the most frequent complaints among individuals who have undergone various cancer treatments. It can also be accompanied by feelings of anxiety, depression, and negativity, or it may increase the mortality rate [6].

There is sufficient evidence to indicate that specific exercise guidelines for cancer patients improve quality of life, physical fitness, and independence in daily activities. In addition, it helps prevent cancer recurrence [7]. Exercise can play an important role in the management of cancer-related fatigue, reduction of pain, improving bone density, improving and maintaining flexibility of tissues, as well as stimulating the bone marrow immune response. The Physical Activity Guidelines recommend 150 minutes of moderate-intensity aerobic exercises spread over 3–5 days. Additionally, twice-weekly resistance training is recommended, ideally engaging major muscle groups [8]. Another useful exercise is yoga; it helps with flexibility and breathing. The choice of exercise should be determined by the patient's specific condition. A patient's response to a specific physical activity may vary due to comorbidities, age-related demographic characteristics, mobility limitations, or therapeutic side effects [9].

Certain exercises should be avoided or adjusted, especially in cases of bone metastases, bone cancer or lung cancer, as the treatment may cause the bones to be more brittle and weaker. Some patients need to avoid resistance and high-impact exercises, which may increase the risk of injury. Conditions such as anemia, characterized by a low red blood cell count, are often a result of treatment and should be considered before initiating a physical activity program [6].

Overall, exercises show clinical effects that can improve cancer-related health outcomes such as fatigue, lymphedema, urinary incontinence, muscle weakness, osteoporosis, and cancer-related obesity. This chapter introduces common cancer-related dysfunctions and outlines the importance of exercises based on evidence among cancer patients.

2. Cancer-related fatigue

The most common issue among cancer patients is fatigue, tiredness, and exhaustion [10]. It is described as a distressing and persistent symptom related to both cancer and its treatments. Cancer-related fatigue (CRF) differs from normal fatigue; it is prolonged, more generalized, not relieved by rest or sleep, and leads to a loss of desire for activities [11]. Most studies reporting cancer prevalence rates found that 65% of individuals complained of fatigue, with figures rising to 80–90% during chemotherapy or radiotherapy [12]. In addition to hormonal therapy, fatigue can result from targeted therapy, immune therapy and surgery. The extent of fatigue from surgery depends on the type of operation, but most people tend to improve with time. Fatigued patients take 2–3 months to return to normal, but for some, it may take longer [11]. Cancer-related fatigue affects many aspects of a patient's life—physically (performance and activities of daily living), psychologically (mood, self-confidence), and socially (social activities, relationships)—and causes impairment in overall quality of life [12].

Assessment of the CRF should be comprehensive. Self-reporting is an efficient and highly recommended method for measuring CRF. Recent studies suggest that the most effective screening tool is a numerical rating scale (10-point rating scale). Patients are asked to score their fatigue level, with 0 indicating no fatigue and 10 indicating the worst possible fatigue [13]. Moreover, contributing factors such as comorbidities, mental and medical status, and other factors like anemia, infection, and conditions such as thyroid, renal, or cardiopulmonary diseases need to be assessed with specific attention as these factors significantly contribute to CRF [11].

Prolonged inactivity can lead to a reduction in musculoskeletal mass and power, psychological well-being, cardiovascular fitness, and activities of daily living [11]. Exercises can be beneficial at different stages of CRF, with no specific form of exercise found to be more beneficial than others. Exercises have not only been found effective in reducing CRF but also in improving cardiovascular fitness, psychological well-being, and quality of life. According to the current exercise guidelines, individuals should engage in 150 minutes per week of aerobic exercises, 2 days per week of resistance training, and flexibility exercises on days when no aerobic or resistance exercise is performed [11].

Resistance exercises not only reduce cancer-related fatigue, but also increase muscle strength, engage large muscle groups, lower blood lipids, optimize immune activity and promote an anti-inflammatory state [11, 14]. Randomized control trials (RCTs) have indicated that both resistance training and endurance exercises are safe and recommended whether performed at high-intensity or low-to-moderate intensity (with 12-week exercising program, twice per week). The exercises targeted large muscle groups with the aim of maximizing improvements in cardiorespiratory fitness; the relative improvements in peakVO2 (15–20%) for high-intensity and low-to-moderate, across different types of cancer diseases [14]. Therefore, combining resistance exercise with aerobic training improves physical functions and reduces chemotherapy related symptoms, including fatigue [15]. In a meta-analysis involving 3254 participants diagnosed with varying cancer types and stages during or after treatment, it was observed that combining resistance exercise with aerobic training at moderate to high intensity for a 6-month follow-up resulted in significantly less decline in cardiorespiratory fitness (ES, 0.14), improved physical functioning (ES, 0.68), reduced nausea and vomiting (ES, 1.00), decreased pain (ES, 0.60), and better outcomes for muscle strength (ES, 0.45) and physical fatigue(ES, 0.51). Additionally, low intensity exercises implemented as a home program prove to be beneficial for women who may be unable or unwilling to adhere to a higher-intensity program [16]. Aerobic training alone has been suggested as a treatment for CRF. As demonstrated in another systematic review comprising 40 trials, aerobic training exercises such as running, swimming, and walking, conducted over a 12-week follow-up, were found to significantly decrease fatigue in cancer survivors (the effect size in EORTC QLQ-C30 fatigue scale was −22.45 and in Liner analog self-assessment scale was −19.00). This positive effect was observed even when the exercise interventions were reported as either moderate to vigorous or low to moderate intensity [17].

For fatigued patients, brisk walking, stationary cycling, or treadmill exercises, along with other exercises, is recommended for at least 30–60 minutes per week. Patients can start their exercise routine with a low intensity, such as 5 minutes per week, and gradually increase up to 30 minutes over the course of a week or month [18]. Walking at a moderate intensity (50–70% of maximum heart rate) during chemotherapy and radiation therapy for breast cancer, starting from 10 to 45 minutes daily, for 4–6 days per week over 6 months, has been shown to reduce CRF and improve quality of life in non-cachectic patients [19].

Yoga exercise is another important intervention for preventing fatigue. A study conducted with breast cancer women shows that yoga, especially with deep breathing exercises, offers symptomatic relief for depression, sleep disorders, and results in a substantial reduction in fatigue. It can include different positions, such as the "Dead Men's Position" ("Shavasana") or "The Lying Butterfly" ("Supta Baddha Konasana").

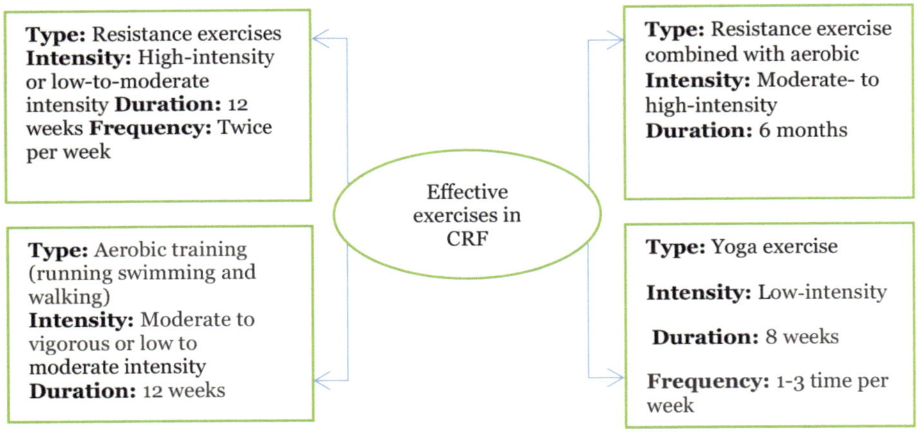

Figure 1.
Exercise recommendation for CRF.

Each of these positions was practiced for up to 7–10 minutes for an eight-week program [18]. Yoga is considered a low-intensity mind-body exercise (BMT). A systematic review and meta-analysis were conducted to evaluate the effects of yoga, Tai chi, and Qigong in alleviating the adverse effects of chemotherapy (breast, lung, and colorectal cancer). Quality of life, fatigue, and the six-minute walk test (6 MWT) were screened. The study found a significant reduction in fatigue among colorectal cancer patients undergoing chemotherapy after MBT interventions. The mean difference was observed in Fatigue: −1.35, 6MWT: −36.05, Quality of life: 3.88 [20]. Long duration of practicing yoga is more beneficial than short term intervention. A meta-analysis evaluated the effect of yoga on cancer-related fatigue in 2183 patients with breast cancer. It was concluded that supervised yoga classes had a significant effect on CRF (SMD = −0.31, 95% CI(−0.52, −0.10)); the eight-week program demonstrated a large effect compared to the six-week program, which had a moderately beneficial effect for 60–90 minutes in each session [21].

Exercises are recommended as a potential treatment for CRF and are supported by strong evidence (**Figure 1**). The patient should be encouraged to initiate physical activity, and the therapist should tailor the intensity and duration of the intervention based on the patient's abilities, as outlined in the program's benefits. However, future research is required to fully understand the factors and practical obstacles that hinder cancer patients from engaging in physical activity both before and after their treatment. Additionally, there is need to develop appropriate guidelines or protocols for CRF. Further studies are needed to assess the effectiveness of yoga exercises in other type of cancer treatments.

3. Lymphedema

Lymphedema, a localized form of tissue swelling, is the accumulation of excessive amounts of interstitial fluid in the tissues, resulting in chronic swelling and other associated symptoms in one or more regions of the body [22]. Lymphedema develops in approximately 20–25% of women after axillary lymph node dissection and about 5% after sentinel lymph node biopsy [23].

Lymphedema can occur during or after many months or years after radiotherapy or immediately following lymph node dissection, significantly impacting people's lives physically, functionally, psychologically, and economically. Patients may report physical effects of the treatment, including swelling, discomfort, and heaviness. Breast cancer-related lymphedema can increase the risk of cellulitis and cause skin and tissue changes, further affecting musculoskeletal issues. For example, trauma to the long thoracic nerve during axillary dissection and lymph node removal can lead to shoulder weakness, resulting in scapular instability due to serratus anterior weakness, frozen shoulder, decreased grip strength, and postural malalignment. The patient may experience changes in daily tasks, such as household chores, self-care tasks, leisure activities, and sleep/rest patterns. This, in turn, can then impact activity, participation, and the overall quality of life [24]. Moreover, it can lead to psychological issues, including changes to sexual drive, body image, energy levels, anxiety, depression, and fear. Breast cancer-related lymphedema may further exacerbate these concerns [25].

The evaluation and examination of lymphatic function starts with patient history, noting any history of trauma, surgery, radiation, chemotherapy, as well as details about the duration, onset, and period of chemotherapy. Furthermore, an examination of skin integrity, a pitting test, circumferential tape measure readings, and bioimpedance spectroscopy (BIS) are conducted [26].

There is currently no cure for lymphedema, and the primary objective of treatment is to restore the lymphedema to the latency stage as much as possible. The gold-standard treatment for lymphedema is the complex decongestive therapy (CDT) protocol, which includes manual lymphatic drainage (MLD), compression therapy, exercises, and skin care. In comprehensive management and rehabilitation, the effectiveness and limitations should be determined by the therapist. The complex decongestive therapy is divided into two stages: the first stage focuses on intensive treatment for reduction, while the second stage is dedicated to long-term management for maintenance. The first stage at the beginning includes a manual lymphatic drainage—a light repetitive stroking massage movement designed to stimulate the lymph nodes and improve their activity. Compression therapy varies depending on the stage of treatment. In the initial stage, low-stretching bandages are used, offering low resting pressure and high working pressure throughout the day. As patients transition from the initial stage to the maintenance stage, compression garments are used during the daytime, providing high resting pressure and low working pressure [27, 28].

Various forms of exercise seem to be safe interventions for treating lymphedema and offer benefits such as improved quality of life, strength, BMI, and decreased pain [29]. The standard guidelines recommend avoiding weight lifting using affected limbs to prevent exacerbations of lymphedema. However, in a controlled trial assessing the effectiveness of weight lifting among 141 breast-cancer survivors with stable arm lymphedema, it was concluded that weight lifting did not significantly alter the severity of lymphedema associated with breast cancer, as measured by displaced water volume (an absolute rise of ≥5 percentage points in the limb volume difference). Additionally, weight lifting resulted in a decreased incidence of exacerbations of lymphedema, reduced symptoms, and increased strength. The exercises consisted of high-frequency dynamic and moderate training, which included a cardiovascular warm-up, abdominal and back exercises, and weight lifting exercises. The upper-body exercises included seated rows, chest press, lateral or front raises, bicep curls, and triceps pushdowns. Additionally, the lower-body exercises included leg press, back extension, leg extension, and leg curl (for a 90-minute session, twice weekly for a year) [30].

The compression bandage must be worn during exercises to avoid lymphatic backflow. This is because the muscle contractions enhance the movement of lymph within lymph vessels, resulting in reduced volume and an increased strength pattern [31]. For example, a study examined the impact of low-intensity strengthening exercises, either associated with or without Complex Physical Therapy (CPT). The exercises, involving the use of a TheraBand, stick, and a little ball, were performed for 10–15 repetitions on 2–3 sets, twice a week over 8 weeks. The study concluded that exercises, whether associated with CPT or not, can be implemented safely and result in similar increases in range of movement and muscle strength without the risk of increasing upper limb volume with edema. Whereas, the mean difference of limb volume reduction after exercising with CPT: 119 mm compared to without CPT: 297 mm [32]. In a single randomized controlled crossover trial, it was found that gynecological cancer-related lower limb lymphedema was significantly reduced after high-load active exercise with compression therapy (AECT) compared to low-load AECT (The mean change (95%CI) of Lower-limb volume; 31.7–93.3 and 19.5–80.6, respectively). The study used the Strength Ergo™240 bicycle ergometer, with durations ranging from 15 to 60 minutes [33]. Another systematic review and meta-analysis evaluated the effects of aerobic, resistance, and mixed exercise on cancer-related lymphedema, specifically determining the need for wearing compression during exercise over a period ranging from 8 weeks to more than 12 weeks. The study observed immediate significant reductions in limb swelling after exercises. However, long-term effect was not found to be significant. The standardized mean differences (SMD) from all analyses were ranging between −0.2 and 0.1 [34].

In addition, stretching and flexibility exercises are strongly recommended to alleviate hypomobility in soft tissues and joints [31]. In addition to deep breathing exercises (abdominal diaphragmatic), they assist in the movement of lymphatic fluid during deep inspiration, maximum expiration, and abdominal contraction [31]. Other interventions to reduce lymphedema are yoga exercises, which have shown positive results in treating breast cancer survivors. In a span of 8–12 weeks, yoga interventions were found to reduce tissue induration in the affected upper arm compared to usual care [35, 36].

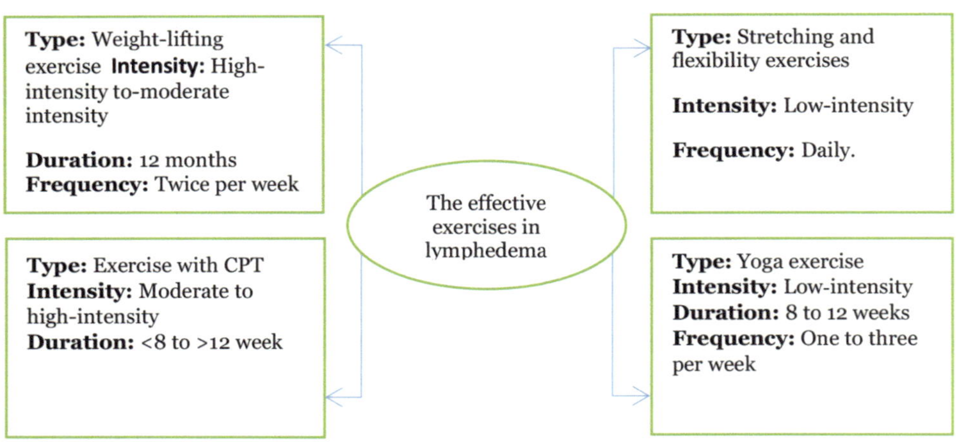

Figure 2.
Exercise recommendation for lymphedema.

Resistance exercises combined with aerobics or yoga with or without CPT may be beneficial and safe to reduce lymphedema (**Figure 2**), but most studies have found that exercises decreased the incidence of exacerbations. Overall, there is insufficient scientific evidence to strongly support this point.

4. Chemotherapy-induced peripheral neuropathy (CIPN)

Approximately 68% of cancer patients experience chemotherapy-induced peripheral neuropathy within the first month of receiving chemotherapy [37]. It is a syndrome characterized by highly distressing symptoms of varying degrees of severity that significantly impact daily functioning [3]. Its presentation varies depending on the type of affected nerve fibers [37]. If sensory nerves are affected, symptoms may include numbness, tingling, stinging, pain, weakness, or burning. Conversely, damage to the motor nerves can cause muscle spasms and muscle wasting, a loss of muscle dexterity and diminished strength. Additionally, damage in the autonomic system may affect and cause autonomic symptoms related to orthostatic hypotension [38].

There are six specific chemotherapy drugs that are more likely to cause peripheral neuropathy, such as platinum-based drugs, taxanes, vinca alkaloids, bortezomib, epothilones, proteasome inhibitors, and immunomodulatory drugs. The mechanisms of these therapeutic drugs are diverse and include both DNA and microtubular targets to arrest cell division and induce cell death. The pathophysiological processes are multifactorial, including oxidative stress, apoptotic mechanisms, altered calcium homeostasis, axon degeneration and membrane remodeling, immune processes and neuro-inflammation [37].

The diagnosis of CIPN should include patient history, current treatments, social history, physical examination, lab tests, electrodiagnostic studies, and nerve biopsy if needed [38].

Exercise may treat or prevent CIPN, as suggested by the RCT study involving 355 patients who received chemotherapy. The study evaluated a standardized, individualized, home-based progressive walking and resistance exercise program compared to those without a standard care control group. Their results stated that exercises can reduce CIPN symptoms of hot or coldness in hands or feet, numbness, and tingling by nearly 0.5 units on the 0–10 scales compared to the participants in the control group. Moreover, the exercise program included low to moderate-intensity home-based walking (60–85% of heart rate reserve) and low to moderately intense resistance exercise (squat, side bend, leg extension, leg curl, chest press, row, calf raise, overhead press, biceps curl, triceps extension) along with four optional band exercises (front raise, lateral raise, internal rotation, external rotation). Participants performed these exercises daily for a 6-week period, with a maximum of 4 sets of 15 repetitions [39]. Furthermore, CIPN symptoms may be better managed effectively in individuals who are younger, fitter, and leaner by utilizing high-intensity aerobic activity (180 minutes per week, 3 times per week) instead of low-intensity exercise (90 minutes per week). This was demonstrated during treatment in 301 women with breast cancer in an RCT [40].

Overall, several clinical trials and studies have demonstrated the potential advantages of various types of exercise and intensities for cancer patients receiving chemotherapy or following chemotherapy who have been diagnosed with CIPN (mixed cancer types and stages and CIPN severity). Balance, walking, resistance, and aerobic

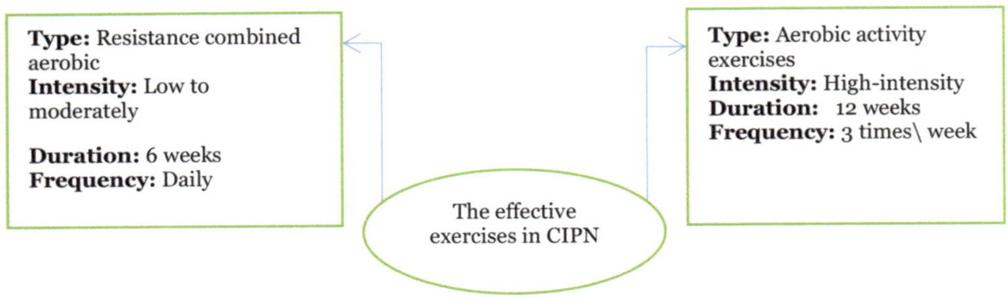

Figure 3.
Exercise recommendation for CIPN.

exercises, or combined exercises (**Figure 3**), provided not only benefits in patients with CIPN but also improved quality of life, Barthel index, the 6-minute walk test (6MWT), balance, and muscle strength [15, 41–44].

5. Urinary incontinence

Urinary incontinence (UI) is an involuntary loss of urine or the inability to control urination. The subtype of UI includes urge urinary incontinence, characterized by involuntary leakage immediately preceded by urgency. It occurs when the bladder contracts abnormally during filling, creating a progressively stronger and undeniable sensation of the need to urinate. Urinary incontinence can be associated with an overactive bladder; individuals may be "at least slightly bothered by frequent urination" and/or experience "leakage related to feeling of urgency". Stress incontinence is involuntary leakage related to physical activity, coughing, or sneezing. It happens due to increased intra-abdominal pressure and when the urethral sphincter is unable to maintain a pressure higher than that exerted on the bladder. Mixed urinary incontinence is characterized by the presence of both stress and urge incontinence [45, 46].

Approximately 34% of women treated for the three main types of gynecologic cancers—cervical, endometrial, and ovarian—complained of urinary incontinence [47]. Additionally, it may occur after prostatectomy or radiation therapy [48], or following surgical treatment of rectal cancer [49]. Furthermore, 38% of cervical cancer survivors report chronic pelvic pain, chronic enteritis, proctitis, cystitis, and tenesmus-associated urinary or fecal urgency as common radiation-related adhesions [50]. The genital system can be impacted during cancer intervention, leading to dyspareunia secondary to menopause, decreased vaginal lubrication from radiation, and vaginal stricture or fibrosis resulting from radiation. Approximately 34–58% of women experience UI, a higher prevalence compared to men [50]. On the other hand, UI is a common problem in patients with early-stage breast cancer receiving neoadjuvant therapy. Approximately 79.8% of women experienced UI before the initiation of systemic therapy in the year following primary treatment, with symptoms related to chemotherapy. Endocrine therapy and adjuvant chemotherapy can exacerbate bladder control problems, hot flashes, and vaginal issues, particularly in older women, and these challenges are sometimes difficult to resolve [51]. There are other factors associated with UI and their impact on quality of life aside from cancer treatment, such as age, menopausal status, body mass index (BMI), race or ethnicity, history of smoking, and parity (0, 1, 2, or $\geq$ 3 births) [52].

The examination for UI includes manual evaluation or electrical devices to assess muscle power, contraction, endurance, and dermatome. The treatment program is determined according to the level of weakness.

The pelvic floor rehabilitation program improves pelvic floor dysfunction and quality of life in gynecological cancer patients. The contractions effectively inhibit detrusor muscle hypertrophy, increasing mechanical pressure on urethra and preventing urinary incontinence. An excellent example of strengthening exercises is Kegel exercises. Studies have demonstrated that the exercises could help prevent cystocele, rectocele, and urinary stress incontinence. However, about 30% of women could not contract the pelvic floor muscles correctly [53]. A Study involving 90 urogynecology women aimed to assess the effects of home-based Kegel exercises in women with stress and mixed urinary incontinence. The study revealed statistically significant improvements in outcomes, including the Incontinence Impact Questionnaire (IIQ-7), Urogenital Distress Inventory (UDI-6), and the Patient Global Impression of Improvement (PGI-I) questions (The mean changes in SUI: 24, 29, 26 and SUI: 9, 11, 14, respectively), after 8 weeks of exercising. The Kegel exercises for stress UI and mixed UI consisted of 10 sets of contractions and 10 repetitions daily for at least 8 weeks [54]. The short duration of exercise, specifically a four-week pelvic floor rehabilitation program (PFRP), involved only one session per day. This program included a second set of 20 to 30 seconds of fast pelvic floor contractions in addition to the first set of longer contractions. The results showed improvements in pelvic floor strength and sexual function (mean difference (MD) =14.22, $t_9 = 2.389$) compared with the non-PFRP group [48]. Another study on pelvic floor muscle contractions, with the goal of holding the contraction for 5 seconds in 3 sets daily over twelve weeks, demonstrated an 80% improvement in UI [55]. Similarly, in a systematic review of 886 patients with pelvic floor dysfunction after gynecological cancer concluded that pelvic floor muscle training (PFMT) with yoga or core exercises was 95% beneficial for sexual function and urinary incontinence [56]. In addition, PFMT significantly improved patient-reported stress incontinence from 1 month to 1 year after prostatectomy [57].

Pelvic floor muscle training could include coordination training, strength training, abdominal and trunk stabilization, or relaxation training, with or without the use of biofeedback, as recommended. The use of biofeedback increases men's ability

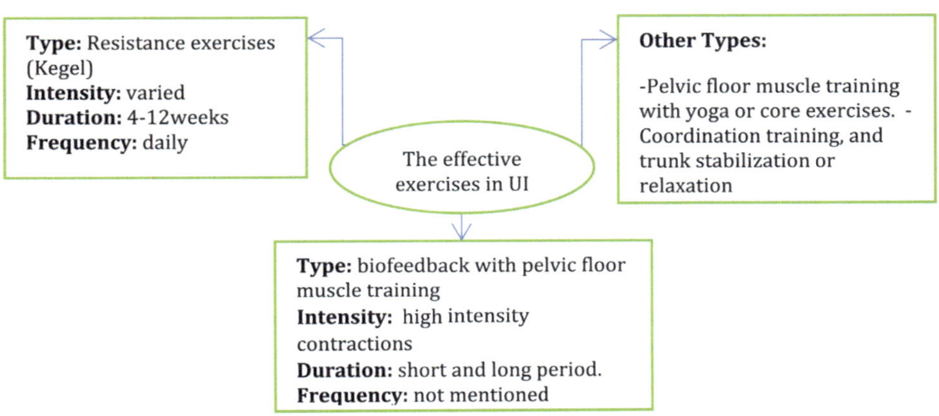

Figure 4.
Exercise recommendation for UI.

to isolate the pelvic floor muscle and differentiate between muscle contraction and relaxation. Studies have indicated that incorporating biofeedback with PFMT during the preoperative and early postoperative period helps expedite the recovery of continence in both the short and long term. These exercises consist of repeated, high-intensity muscle contractions [58]. Research is needed to determine the most effective treatment, as there is no established exercise protocol for urinary incontinence in cancer patients. The duration, intensity, and frequency varied, but they contributed to improving the UI. Most studies assessed the effectiveness of PFMT without specifying the type of exercises performed. Overall PFMT is recommended for cancer patients (**Figure 4**).

6. Osteoporosis

Osteoporosis is essentially the loss of bone mass in the trabecular region, leading to diminished density and an increased risk of fractures. It increases the risk of mortality and affects quality of life. All cancers can have significant negative effects on the skeleton through various mechanisms, either directly impacted by cancer cells or due to cancer treatments, including chemotherapy, corticosteroids, aromatase inhibitors, hormonal therapy such as tamoxifen for women with breast cancer, and androgen deprivation therapy for patients with prostate cancer [59]. Additionally, these effects are observed in gastric cancer patients who underwent gastrectomy [60] and gynecological cancer [61]. Besides, older patients or postmenopausal women are at a greater risk of bone loss and fractures compared to premenopausal women. Metastatic bone involvement is one of the complications of solid tumors and can affect the spine, pelvis, skull, ribs, proximal humerus, and femur [60].

Fractures caused by osteoporosis are termed fragility fractures. Common sites include the wrist and hip, often resulting from falls impacting either on an outstretched hand or directly onto the hip. However, the most common fracture occurs in the vertebral region. This fracture typically develops silently, accompanied by changes in posture, poor mechanics, repeated bending, and end-range forces. Exercises can contribute to improving bone remodeling, matrix mineralization, and bone marrow health. However, health professionals should carefully assess the risk of bone fragility and metastatic cancer, apply safe principles for alignment, and individualize the exercise program to prevent complications [60, 61]. Contraindications should also be taken into account.

Exercises are safe for cancer patients with osteoporosis and show effectiveness in maintaining or improving bone health during or after cancer treatment. Additionally, they help prevent comorbidities related to cancer such as obesity, cardiovascular disease, and type 2 diabetes [62]. This was supported by a 26-week study on female cancer survivors involving combined aerobic and resistance training, which reported significant improvements in bone mass density (BMD) at the spine (2.5%), hip (1.5%), and whole body (2.0%) as investigated using dual-energy X-ray absorptiometry (DXA). The exercises were performed 3 days per week, with sessions consisting of 20 minutes of cardiorespiratory training, 25 minutes of circuit-style resistance training, and 15 minutes of abdominal exercises and stretching [61]. Strengthening and weight training exercises, when combined with medication such as risedronate, calcium, and vitamin D, have been found to have effects and may prevent the loss of BMD at the femoral neck (SMD = +0.29%), total hip (SMD = +0.34%), spine (SMD = +0.23%), total radius (SMD = +0.30%)

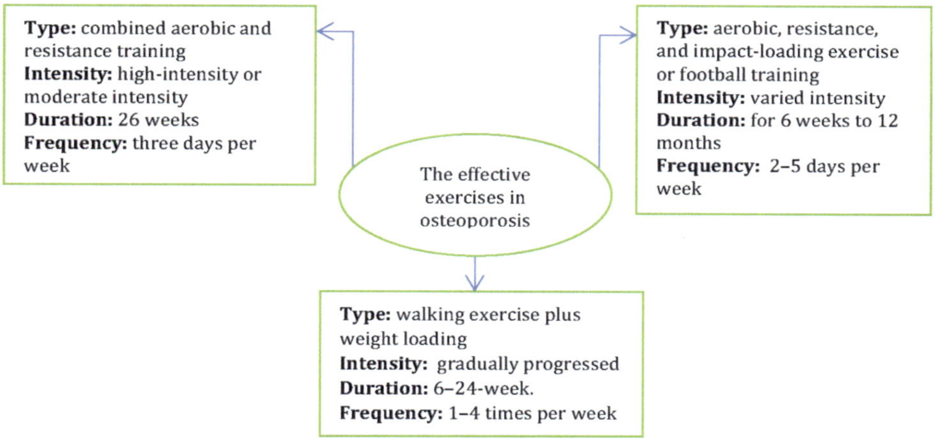

Figure 5.
Exercise recommendation for osteoporosis.

in postmenopausal women [63]. On the other hand, aerobic weight-loaded exercise did not show significant changes in serum osteocalcin, serum NTX, or lean muscle mass among women within 2 years of menopause who had completed adjuvant chemotherapy and adjuvant endocrine therapy. The participants engaged in a 6–24-week supervised walking exercise plus weight loading (1–4 times per week, with progressively increased weight). At the end of the study, it was suggested that a weight-loaded aerobic exercise intervention has the potential to maintain bone mass in women at risk for bone loss [64].

Only 41.9% of men with prostate cancer undergoing androgen deprivation therapy engage in the recommended amount of exercise, indicating a higher level of inactivity [65]. The most crucial aspect is to develop a habit for exercising. Patients may be advised to start with brief workouts (15 minutes per day, several times per week) before establishing a routine [66]. Nine RCTs provided a combination of aerobic, resistance, and impact-loading exercise or an hour-long football training lasting for 6 weeks to 12 months, with varied intensity and frequency (2–5 days per week). Participants could safely engage in exercise programs to preserve bone health and successfully exercise as a crucial part of their lifestyle. The findings demonstrate that exercises are relatively feasible and safe, and such exercises have the potential to reduce the risk of accidental falls, fractures, and associated morbidity and mortality rates. Moreover, this review shows a higher adherence rate from 43% to 96.3% and the retention rate from 71.9–100% in experimental exercise programs [67].

All types of exercise contribute to improving bone density and reducing risk of falls, injuries, with a significant impact on health-related quality of life. Regular exercise not only reduces mortality but should also be adopted as a long-term lifestyle habit (**Figure 5**).

7. Obesity-related cancer

Many cancer patients experience weight gain after diagnosis, which is more common in those undergoing chemotherapy. Some patients also complain of loss of muscle mass and concomitant gain of adipose tissue, a condition referred to as cachexia [68]. Obesity increases the risk of cancer, with more than 40,000 cancer diagnoses each year attributed to obesity [69]. It is also linked to poorer cancer outcomes in breast, prostate, and colorectal cancers. More than two-thirds of survivors of breast, prostate, gynecologic, pancreatic, colorectal, ovarian cancer, and hematologic malignancies are overweight or obese [70]. Obesity in cancer survivors is a risk factor for developing comorbidities, such as heart disease, cerebrovascular disease, and diabetes [71]. Overweight is categorized as a BMI greater than or equal to 25, and obesity is categorized as a BMI greater than 30 [68].

The American Society of Clinical Oncology (ASCO) is committed to reducing the impact of obesity on cancer survivors and encourages participation in weight loss programs after the completion of adjuvant chemotherapy and radiotherapy [68]. A reduction in obesity through physical activity can improve insulin sensitivity, decrease circulating glucose and insulin levels, improve immune surveillance and recirculation of immunoglobulin, neutrophils, cytotoxic T cells, and immature B cells, and improve blood lipids and metabolic health [72]. Research has shown that weight loss strategies combining nutrition, physical activity, and psychological support can enhance the quality of life and lower the BMI of individuals who have survived breast cancer [73, 74]. For example, a study involving 351 survivors of breast cancer with overweight or obesity for a 52-week treatment program concluded that both increased physical activity and calorie restriction may lead to more significant weight loss (mean change: −6.68 kg) compared to caloric restriction (mean change: −5.39 kg) or increased physical activity (mean change: −0.06 kg) alone [74]. *Another systematic review and meta-analysis found that various types of exercises improved cardiorespiratory fitness* (SMD = 0.44), *reducing bodyweight* (SMD = 0.11) *and waist circumference* (SMD = 0.22) *in cancer patients. The exercises included aerobics, resistance training (for the large muscles of the upper and lower limbs), yoga, walking, cycling, tai chi chuan, and cycling exercises, performed for 30 to 60 minutes, at 50–60% of one repetition maximum, for two to three sets. The frequency ranged from two to five times per week for a duration of 3 months to 2 years* [75]. On the other hand, a few other studies found that exercise had only a limited impact on body composition, such as BMI, in obese or overweight breast cancer survivors [76, 77].

Generally, physical exercise is associated with weight reduction, a lower BMI, a lower percentage of body fat, and an increase in the quality of life. It is recommended either alone or in combination with other interventions. Future studies, including other types of cancer, are needed (**Figure 6**).

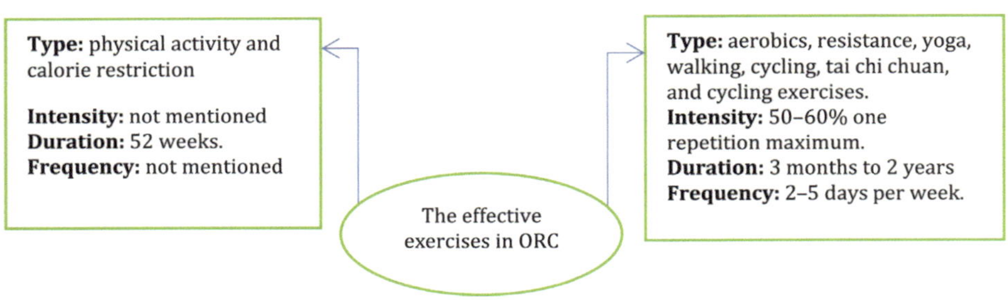

Figure 6.
Exercise recommendation for obesity related cancer.

8. Conclusions

Cancer patients suffer from multiple symptoms during treatments or as side effects after treatment. Physical activity helps improve quality of life, reduce mortality, and prevent the recurrence of cancer. There are no specific types or frequency that should be followed; the exercise program built up depends on the patient's tolerance and other factors. In this chapter the evidence showed different effectiveness of exercises as follows:

The current exercise guidelines indicate that cancer patients should engage in 150 minutes of moderate-intensity resistance, aerobic, and flexibility exercises.

All studies demonstrate a significant effect of exercises of all types on improving fatigue, cardiovascular fitness, and other aspects related to quality of life. A longer duration of intervention is better than a short period.

Exercises are safe for lymphedema patients and help prevent exacerbations, but weight lifting or combined aerobics showed immediate effects after exercises in reducing swelling. However, there was no significant alteration in the severity of lymphedema whether associated with CPT or not. Only one study related to gynecological cancer-related lower limb lymphedema shows the opposite.

Balance, walking, resistance, and aerobic exercise or combined exercises are recommended for patients with CIPN.

The pelvic floor rehabilitation program, especially Kegel exercises, is important for cancer patients with urinary incontinence or sexual dysfunction of both genders. Using biofeedback with pelvic floor muscle training is effective as a short- or long-term intervention.

Aerobic and resistance training are safe for cancer patients with osteoporosis and help prevent the loss of BMD in postmenopausal women or prostate cancer patients with ADT.

Exercises alone or in combination with other interventions are recommended, but studies have shown a limited impact on body composition and BMI.

Acknowledgements

I would like to express my deepest gratitude to the head of holistic care in Sultan Qaboos comprehensive cancer care and research center for moral support and inspiration.

Author details

Hajer Alhinai
Sultan Qaboos Comprehensive Cancer Care and Research Center (SQCCCRC), Muscat, Oman

*Address all correspondence to: h.alhinai@cccrc.gov.om

References

[1] Siegel RL, Miller KD, Wagle NS, Jemal A. Cancer statistics, 2023. CA: A Cancer Journal for Clinicians. 2023;**73**(1):17-48. DOI: 10.3322/caac.21763

[2] Miller KD, Siegel RL, Lin CC, Mariotto AB, Kramer JL, Rowland JH, et al. Cancer treatment and survivorship statistics, 2016. CA: A Cancer Journal for Clinicians. 2016;**66**(4):271-289. DOI: 10.3322/caac.21349. Epub 2016 Jun 2

[3] Brzeziński K. Chemotherapy-induced polyneuropathy. Part I. Pathophysiology. Contemporary Oncology (Pozn). 2012;**16**(1):72-78. DOI: 10.5114/wo.2012.27341. Epub 2012 Feb 29

[4] Chaput G, Regnier L. Radiotherapy: Clinical pearls for primary care. Canadian Family Physician. 2021;**67**(10):753-757. DOI: 10.46747/cfp.6710753

[5] Lovelace DL, McDaniel LR, Golden D. Long-term effects of breast Cancer surgery, treatment, and survivor care. Journal of Midwifery & Women's Health. 2019;**64**(6):713-724. DOI: 10.1111/jmwh.13012. Epub 2019 Jul 19

[6] Campbell KL, Winters-Stone KM, et al. Exercise guidelines for Cancer survivors: Consensus statement from international multidisciplinary roundtable. Medicine and Science in Sports and Exercise. 2019;**51**(11):2375-2390. DOI: 10.1249/MSS.0000000000002116

[7] COSA Exercise and Cancer Group Executive Committee. Clinical oncology Society of Australia position statement on exercise in cancer care. The Medical Journal of Australia. 2019;**210**(1):54-54.e1. DOI: 10.5694/mja2.12039. Epub 2018 Dec 7

[8] Schmitz KH, Campbell AM, et al. Exercise is medicine in oncology: Engaging clinicians to help patients move through cancer. CA: A Cancer Journal for Clinicians. 2019;**69**(6):468-484. DOI: 10.3322/caac.21579. Epub 2019 Oct 16

[9] Parker NH, Arlinghaus KR, Johnston CA. Integrating physical activity into clinical Cancer care. American Journal of Lifestyle Medicine. 2018;**12**:220-223. DOI: 10.1177/1559827618759478

[10] Mock V, Atkinson A, Barsevick A, Cella D, Cimprich B, Cleeland C, et al. National Comprehensive Cancer Network. NCCN practice guidelines for Cancer-related fatigue. Oncology (Williston Park). 2000;**14**(11A):151-161

[11] Fabi A, Bhargava R, Fatigoni S, Guglielmo M, Horneber M, Roila F, et al. Electronic address: clinicalguidelines@esmo.org. Cancer-related fatigue: ESMO clinical practice guidelines for diagnosis and treatment. Annals of Oncology. 2020;**31**(6):713-723. DOI: 10.1016/j.annonc.2020.02.016. Epub 2020 Mar 12

[12] Bower JE, Ganz PA, Desmond KA, Bernaards C, Rowland JH, Meyerowitz BE, et al. Fatigue in long-term breast carcinoma survivors: A longitudinal investigation. Cancer. 2006;**106**(4):751-758. DOI: 10.1002/cncr.21671

[13] Fisher MI, Davies C, Lacy H, Doherty D. Oncology section EDGE task force on Cancer: Measures of Cancer-related fatigue—A systematic review. Rehabilitation Oncology. 2018;**36**(2):93-105. DOI: 10.1097/01.REO.0000000000000124

[14] Kampshoff CS, Chinapaw MJ, Brug J, Twisk JW, Schep G, Nijziel MR,

et al. Randomized controlled trial of the effects of high intensity and low-to-moderate intensity exercise on physical fitness and fatigue in cancer survivors: Results of the resistance and endurance exercise after ChemoTherapy (REACT) study. BMC Medicine. 2015;**13**:275. DOI: 10.1186/s12916-015-0513-2

[15] Courneya KS, Segal RJ, et al. Effects of aerobic and resistance exercise in breast cancer patients receiving adjuvant chemotherapy: A multicenter randomized controlled trial. Journal of Clinical Oncology. 2007;**25**(28):4396-4404. DOI: 10.1200/JCO.2006.08.2024. Epub 2007 Sep 4

[16] van Waart H, Stuiver MM, et al. Effect of low-intensity physical activity and moderate- to high-intensity physical exercise during adjuvant chemotherapy on physical fitness, fatigue, and chemotherapy completion rates: Results of the PACES randomized clinical trial. Journal of Clinical Oncology. 2015;**33**(17):1918-1927. DOI: 10.1200/JCO.2014.59.1081. Epub 2015 Apr 27

[17] Mishra SI, Scherer RW, Geigle PM, Berlanstein DR, Topaloglu O, Gotay CC, et al. Exercise interventions on health-related quality of life for cancer survivors. Cochrane Database of Systematic Reviews. 2012;**2012**(8):CD007566. DOI: 10.1002/14651858.CD007566.pub2

[18] Eidenberger M. Physiotherapeutic management in breast cancer patients. In: Breast Cancer Updates. IntechOpen; 3 May 2023. Crossref. DOI: 10.5772/intechopen.108946

[19] Mock V, Pickett M, Ropka ME, Muscari Lin E, Stewart KJ, Rhodes VA, et al. Fatigue and quality of life outcomes of exercise during cancer treatment. Cancer Practice. 2001;**9**(3):119-127. DOI: 10.1046/j.1523-5394.2001.009003119.x

[20] Bailey LE, Morris MA. Mind-body therapies adjuvant to chemotherapy improve quality of life and fatigue in top cancers: A systematic review and meta-analysis. Complementary Therapies in Clinical Practice. 2023;**54**:101811. DOI: 10.1016/j.ctcp.2023.101811. Epub ahead of print

[21] Dong B, Xie C, Jing X, Lin L, Tian L. Yoga has a solid effect on cancer-related fatigue in patients with breast cancer: A meta-analysis. Breast Cancer Research and Treatment. 2019;**177**(1):5-16. DOI: 10.1007/s10549-019-05278-w. Epub 2019 May 24

[22] Casley-Smith JR, Gaffney RM. Excess plasma proteins as a cause of chronic inflammation and lymphodema: Quantitative electron microscopy. The Journal of Pathology. 1981;**133**(3):243-272. DOI: 10.1002/path.1711330307

[23] Greene AK, Goss JA. Diagnosis and staging of lymphedema. Seminars in Plastic Surgery. 2018;**32**(1):12-16. DOI: 10.1055/s-0038-1635117. Epub 2018 Apr 9

[24] Ververs JM, Roumen RM, Vingerhoets AJ, et al. Risk, severity and predictors of physical and psychological morbidity after axillary lymph node dissection for breast cancer. European Journal of Cancer. 2001;**37**(8):991-999

[25] Shih YC, Xu Y, Cormier JN, Giordano S, Ridner SH, Buchholz TA, et al. Incidence, treatment costs, and complications of lymphedema after breast cancer Among women of working age: A 2-year follow-up study. Journal of Clinical Oncology. 2009;**27**(12):2007-2014. DOI: 10.1200/JCO.2008.18.3517. Epub 2009 Mar 16

[26] Shahpar H et al. Risk factors of lymph Edema in breast Cancer patients.

International Journal of Breast Cancer. 2013;**2013**(Article ID 641818):7. DOI: 10.1155/2013/641818

[27] Huang TW, Tseng SH, et al. Effects of manual lymphatic drainage on breast cancer-related lymphedema: A systematic review and meta-analysis of randomized controlled trials. World Journal of Surgical Oncology. 2013;**11**:15. DOI: 10.1186/1477-7819-11-15

[28] Tzani I, Tsichlaki M, Zerva E, Papathanasiou G, Dimakakos E. Physiotherapeutic rehabilitation of lymphedema: State-of-the-art. Lymphology. 2018;**51**(1):1-12

[29] Panchik D, Masco S, Zinnikas P, Hillriegel B, Lauder T, Suttmann E, et al. Effect of exercise on breast Cancer-related lymphedema: What the lymphatic surgeon needs to know. Journal of Reconstructive Microsurgery. 2019;**35**(1):37-45. DOI: 10.1055/s-0038-1660832. Epub 2018 Jun 23

[30] Baumann FT, Reike A, Reimer V, Schumann M, Hallek M, Taaffe DR, et al. Effects of physical exercise on breast cancer-related secondary lymphedema: A systematic review. Breast Cancer Research and Treatment. 2018;**170**(1):1-13. DOI: 10.1007/s10549-018-4725-y. Epub 2018 Feb 22

[31] Kisner C, Colby L, Borstad J. Therapeutic Exercise: Foundations and Techniques, 7e. McGraw Hill; 2018. Available from: https://fadavispt.mhmedical.com/content.aspx?bookid=2262&sectionid=175446320

[32] Luz RPC, Simao Haddad CA, Rizzi SKLA, Elias S, Nazario ACP, Facina G. Complex therapy physical alone or associated with strengthening exercises in patients with lymphedema after breast Cancer treatment: A controlled clinical trial. Asian Pacific Journal of Cancer Prevention. 2018;**19**(5):1405-1410. DOI: 10.22034/APJCP.2018.19.5.1405

[33] Fukushima T, Tsuji T, Sano Y, Miyata C, Kamisako M, Hohri H, et al. Immediate effects of active exercise with compression therapy on lower-limb lymphedema. Supportive Care in Cancer. 2017;**25**(8):2603-2610. DOI: 10.1007/s00520-017-3671-2. Epub 2017 Apr 6

[34] Singh B, Disipio T, Peake J, Hayes SC. Systematic review and Meta-analysis of the effects of exercise for those with Cancer-related lymphedema. Archives of Physical Medicine and Rehabilitation. 2016;**97**(2):302-315.e13. DOI: 10.1016/j.apmr.2015.09.012. Epub 2015 Oct 9

[35] Saraswathi V, Latha S, Niraimathi K, Vidhubala E. Managing lymphedema, increasing range of motion, and quality of life through yoga therapy among breast Cancer survivors: A systematic review. International Journal of Yoga. 2021;**14**(1):3-17. DOI: 10.4103/ijoy.IJOY_73_19. Epub 2021 Feb 5

[36] Loudon A, Barnett T, Piller N, Immink MA, Williams AD. Yoga management of breast cancer-related lymphoedema: A randomised controlled pilot-trial. BMC Complementary and Alternative Medicine. 2014;**14**:214. DOI: 10.1186/1472-6882-14-214

[37] Starobova H, Vetter I. Pathophysiology of chemotherapy-induced peripheral neuropathy. Frontiers in Molecular Neuroscience. 2017;**10**:174. DOI: 10.3389/fnmol.2017.00174

[38] Kraychete DC, Sakata RK. Painful peripheral neuropathies. Revista Brasileira de Anestesiologia. 2011;**61**(5):641-658, 351-360. English, Portuguese, Spanish. DOI: 10.1016/S0034-7094(11)70075-7

[39] Kleckner IR, Kamen C, Gewandter JS, Mohile NA, Heckler CE, Culakova E, et al. Effects of exercise during chemotherapy on chemotherapy-induced peripheral neuropathy: A multicenter, randomized controlled trial. Supportive Care in Cancer. 2018;**26**(4):1019-1028. DOI: 10.1007/s00520-017-4013-0. Epub 2017 Dec 14

[40] Courneya KS, McKenzie DC, Mackey JR, Gelmon K, Friedenreich CM, Yasui Y, et al. Subgroup effects in a randomised trial of different types and doses of exercise during breast cancer chemotherapy. British Journal of Cancer. 2014;**111**(9):1718-1725. DOI: 10.1038/bjc.2014.466. Epub 2014 Aug 21

[41] Zhang S. Chemotherapy-induced peripheral neuropathy and rehabilitation: A review. Seminars in Oncology. 2021;**48**(3):193-207. DOI: 10.1053/j.seminoncol.2021.09.004. Epub 2021 Sep 22

[42] Guo S, Han W, Wang P, Wang X, Fang X. Effects of exercise on chemotherapy-induced peripheral neuropathy in cancer patients: A systematic review and meta-analysis. Journal of Cancer Survivorship. 2023;**17**(2):318-331. DOI: 10.1007/s11764-022-01182-3. Epub 2022 Feb 11

[43] Kanzawa-Lee GA, Larson JL, Resnicow K, Smith EML. Exercise effects on chemotherapy-induced peripheral neuropathy: A comprehensive integrative review. Cancer Nursing. 2020;**43**(3):E172-E185. DOI: 10.1097/NCC.0000000000000801

[44] Diotti D, Puce L, Mori L, Trompetto C, Saretti E, Contenti C, et al. The role of physical activity against chemotherapy-induced peripheral neuropathy: A narrative review. Exploration of Neuroprotective Therapy. 2022;**2**:87-99

[45] Chung CP, Behrendt C, Wong L, Flores S, Mortimer JE. Serial assessment of urinary incontinence in breast Cancer survivors undergoing (neo) adjuvant therapy. Journal of the National Comprehensive Cancer Network. 2020;**18**(6):712-716. DOI: 10.6004/jnccn.2020.7535

[46] Ghaderi F, Oskouei AE. Physiotherapy for women with stress urinary incontinence: A review article. Journal of Physical Therapy Science. 2014;**26**(9):1493-1499. DOI: 10.1589/jpts.26.1493. Epub 2014 Sep 17

[47] Skjeldestad FE, Hagen B. Long-term consequences of gynecological cancer treatment on urinary incontinence: A population-based cross-sectional study. Acta Obstetricia et Gynecologica Scandinavica. 2008;**87**(4):469-475. DOI: 10.1080/00016340801948326

[48] Yang EJ, Lim JY, Rah UW, Kim YB. Effect of a pelvic floor muscle training program on gynecologic cancer survivors with pelvic floor dysfunction: A randomized controlled trial. Gynecologic Oncology. 2012;**125**(3):705-711. DOI: 10.1016/j.ygyno.2012.03.045. Epub 2012 Apr 1

[49] Wallner C, Lange MM, Bonsing BA, Maas CP, Wallace CN, Dabhoiwala NF, et al. Cooperative clinical investigators of the Dutch Total Mesorectal excision trial. Causes of fecal and urinary incontinence after total mesorectal excision for rectal cancer based on cadaveric surgery: A study from the cooperative clinical investigators of the Dutch total mesorectal excision trial. Journal of Clinical Oncology. 2008;**26**(27):4466-4472. DOI: 10.1200/JCO.2008.17.3062

[50] Glare PA, Davies PS, Finlay E, Gulati A, Lemanne D, Moryl N, et al. Pain in cancer survivors. Journal of

Clinical Oncology. 2014;**32**(16):1739-1747. DOI: 10.1200/JCO.2013.52.4629. Epub 2014 May 5

[51] Ganz PA, Petersen L, Bower JE, Crespi CM. Impact of adjuvant endocrine therapy on quality of life and symptoms: Observational data over 12 months from the mind-body study. Journal of Clinical Oncology. 2016;**34**(8):816-824. DOI: 10.1200/JCO.2015.64.3866. Epub 2016 Jan 19

[52] Wojcik M, Jarzabek-Bielecka G, Merks P, Plagens-Rotman K, Pisarska-Krawczyk M, Kedzia W, et al. The role of visceral therapy, Kegel's muscle, core stability and diet in pelvic support disorders and urinary incontinence – Including sexological aspects and the role of physiotherapy and osteopathy. Ginekologia Polska. 2022;**93**(12):1018-1027. DOI: 10.5603/GP.a2022.0136

[53] Huang YC, Chang KV. Kegel Exercises. In: StatPearls. Treasure Island (FL): StatPearls Publishing; 2023

[54] Cavkaytar S, Kokanali MK, Topcu HO, Aksakal OS, Doğanay M. Effect of home-based Kegel exercises on quality of life in women with stress and mixed urinary incontinence. Journal of Obstetrics and Gynaecology. 2015;**35**(4):407-410. DOI: 10.3109/01443615.2014.960831. Epub 2014 Sep 29

[55] Rutledge TL, Rogers R, Lee SJ, Muller CY. A pilot randomized control trial to evaluate pelvic floor muscle training for urinary incontinence among gynecologic cancer survivors. Gynecologic Oncology. 2014;**132**(1):154-158. DOI: 10.1016/j.ygyno.2013.10.024. Epub 2013 Oct 29

[56] Brennen R, Lin KY, Denehy L, Frawley HC. The effect of pelvic floor muscle interventions on pelvic floor dysfunction after Gynecological Cancer treatment: A systematic review. Physical Therapy. 2020;**100**(8):1357-1371. DOI: 10.1093/ptj/pzaa081

[57] Xin L, Li M, Pan M. The therapeutic effect of pelvic floor muscle training on stress urinary incontinence following prostatectomy: A systematic review and meta-analysis. Translational Andrology and Urology. 2023;**12**(7):1155-1166. DOI: 10.21037/tau-23-337. Epub 2023 Jul 24

[58] Huri M, Akel BS, Sahin S. Rehabilitation of patients with prostate cancer [Internet]. In: Prostate Cancer - Leading-edge Diagnostic Procedures and Treatments. InTech; 2016. DOI: 10.5772/63989

[59] Drake MT. Osteoporosis and cancer. Current Osteoporosis Reports. 2013;**11**(3):163-170. DOI: 10.1007/s11914-013-0154-3

[60] Avancini A, Benato G, at al. Exercise and bone health in Cancer: Enemy or ally? Cancers (Basel). 2022;**14**(24):6078. DOI: 10.3390/cancers14246078

[61] Almstedt HC, Grote S, et al. Combined aerobic and resistance training improves bone health of female cancer survivors. Bone Reports. 2016;**5**:274-279. DOI: 10.1016/j.bonr.2016.09.003

[62] Winters-Stone KM, Schwartz A, Nail LM. A review of exercise interventions to improve bone health in adult cancer survivors. Journal of Cancer Survivorship. 2010;**4**(3):187-201. DOI: 10.1007/s11764-010-0122-1. Epub 2010 Apr 7

[63] Waltman NL, Twiss JJ, Ott CD, Gross GJ, Lindsey AM, Moore TE, et al. The effect of weight training on bone

mineral density and bone turnover in postmenopausal breast cancer survivors with bone loss: A 24-month randomized controlled trial. Osteoporosis International. 2010;**21**(8):1361-1369. DOI: 10.1007/s00198-009-1083-y. Epub 2009 Oct 3

[64] Knobf MT, Insogna K, DiPietro L, Fennie C, Thompson AS. An aerobic weight-loaded pilot exercise intervention for breast cancer survivors: Bone remodeling and body composition outcomes. Biological Research for Nursing. 2008;**10**(1):34-43. DOI: 10.1177/1099800408320579

[65] Chipperfield K, Fletcher J, et al. Factors associated with adherence to physical activity guidelines in patients with prostate cancer. Psycho-Oncology. 2013;**22**(11):2478-2486. DOI: 10.1002/pon.3310. Epub 2013 Jun 7

[66] Pelman R, Elterman D. Lifestyle and disease, male health and risks. Revista Médica Clínica Las Condes. 2014;**25**:25-29. DOI: 10.1016/S0716-8640(14)70006-9

[67] Cagliari M, Bressi B, et al. Feasibility and safety of physical exercise to preserve bone health in men with prostate Cancer receiving androgen deprivation therapy: A systematic review. Physical Therapy. 2022;**102**(3):pzab288. DOI: 10.1093/ptj/pzab288

[68] Ligibel JA, Alfano CM, et al. American Society of Clinical Oncology position statement on obesity and cancer. Journal of Clinical Oncology. 2014;**32**(31):3568-3574. DOI: 10.1200/JCO.2014.58.4680. Epub 2014 Oct 1

[69] Finkelstein EA, Trogdon JG, Cohen JW, Dietz W. Annual medical spending attributable to obesity: Payer-and service-specific estimates. Health Affairs (Millwood). 2009;**28**(5):w822-w831. DOI: 10.1377/hlthaff.28.5.w822. Epub 2009 Jul 27

[70] Blanchard CM, Courneya KS, Stein K, American Cancer Society's SCS-II. Cancer survivors' adherence to lifestyle behavior recommendations and associations with health-related quality of life: Results from the American Cancer Society's SCS-II. Journal of Clinical Oncology. 2008;**26**(13):2198-2204. DOI: 10.1200/JCO.2007.14.6217

[71] Travis LB, Demark Wahnefried W, Allan JM, Wood ME, Ng AK. Aetiology, genetics and prevention of secondary neoplasms in adult cancer survivors. Nature Reviews. Clinical Oncology. 2013;**10**(5):289-301. DOI: 10.1038/nrclinonc.2013.41. Epub 2013 Mar 26

[72] Larson EA, Dalamaga M, Magkos F. The role of exercise in obesity-related cancers: Current evidence and biological mechanisms. Seminars in Cancer Biology. 2023;**91**:16-26. DOI: 10.1016/j.semcancer.2023.02.008. Epub 2023 Mar 5

[73] Soares Falcetta F, de Araújo Vianna Träsel H, de Almeida FK, et al. Effects of physical exercise after treatment of early breast cancer: systematic review and meta-analysis. Breast Cancer Research and Treatment. 2018;**170**:455-476. DOI: 10.1007/s10549-018-4786-y

[74] Brown JC, Sarwer DB, Troxel AB, et al. A randomized trial of exercise and diet on body composition in survivors of breast cancer with overweight or obesity. Breast Cancer Research and Treatment. 2021;**189**:145-154

[75] Joaquim A, Leão I, et al. Impact of physical exercise programs in breast cancer survivors on health-related quality of life, physical fitness, and body composition: Evidence from systematic reviews and meta-analyses.

Front. Oncologia. 2022;**12**:955505. DOI: 10.3389/fonc.2022.955505

[76] Murtezani A, Ibraimi Z, Bakalli A, Krasniqi S, Disha ED, Kurtishi I. The effect of aerobic exercise on quality of life among breast cancer survivors: A randomized controlled trial. Journal of Cancer Research and Therapeutics. 1900;**10**(3):658-664

[77] Singh B, Spence RR, Steele ML, Sandler CX, Peake JM, Hayes SC. A systematic review and meta-analysis of the safety, feasibility, and effect of exercise in women with stage ii+ breast cancer. Archives of Physical Medicine and Rehabilitation. 2018;**99**(12):2621-2636. DOI: 10.1016/j.apmr.2018.03.026

Section 3

New Applications of Exercise Medicine

Chapter 7

A Healthy Life with Self-Natural Posture Exercise

Yongsuk Seo and Dae Taek Lee

Abstract

This chapter explores the effectiveness of the Self-Natural Posture Exercise (SNPE) program for individuals with chronic pain and musculoskeletal conditions. SNPE emphasizes self-regulation and natural postural correction as a unique approach to rehabilitation. Within this chapter, several studies show positive effects on physical self-concept, pain reduction, and overall health across diverse populations. It has been particularly beneficial for women with chronic low back pain, adolescents, and individuals with various musculoskeletal disorders. Research also explores its impact on energy expenditure, exercise intensity, and pain-related factors, shedding light on its mechanisms and outcomes. The SNPE program demonstrates effectiveness for chronic pain and musculoskeletal conditions across diverse populations. In a 12-week study, significant improvements in muscle power, flexibility, and pain reduction were revealed. Previous research showed a positive impact on the correction of forward head posture, relief from various pains, and improvement in pelvic alignment. SNPE also prevented scoliosis in adolescents and adapted to different energy expenditure levels. This chapter highlights the innovative and impactful nature of SNPE in addressing chronic pain and facilitating rehabilitation across diverse populations. SNPE goes beyond pain management, actively enhancing overall physical well-being and offering promising solutions for various musculoskeletal challenges across a broad demographic spectrum.

Keywords: Self-Natural Posture Exercise (SNPE), chronic pain, fitness, functional movement, pain perception

1. Introduction

In recent years, there has been a growing emphasis within the fields of rehabilitation and exercise science on incorporating innovative and holistic approaches to promote health and well-being [1]. The concept of wellness encompasses various dimensions of an individual's health, including physical, intellectual, emotional, social, spiritual, vocational, financial, and environmental aspects. It reflects a dynamic and evolving process influenced by the interplay of physical, mental, social, and environmental factors. The ultimate objective extends beyond the mere absence of illness to attain a state of overall health and happiness [2].

IntechOpen

Within this evolving setting, the Self-Natural Posture Exercise, known as SNPE, program has emerged as a promising method for addressing various aspects of chronic pain and musculoskeletal conditions. This introductory chapter aims to explores the multifaceted effects of SNPE on physical self-concept, perceived pain reduction, and overall health outcomes in individuals facing chronic pain and musculoskeletal issues. The rationale for investigating SNPE in the context of chronic pain lies in its unique emphasis on self-regulation and natural postural correction [3].

Chronic pain, a complex phenomenon with psychological and emotional scope, significantly influence physical well-being [3, 4]. SNPE, as a self-directed exercise program, offers a distinctive approach to addressing challenges associated with chronic pain by encouraging active individual participation in their therapy [5]. Subsequent chapters examine a diverse range of studies analyzing the impact of SNPE on specific aspects of chronic pain and musculoskeletal conditions. These studies provide valuable insights into the potential of SNPE as an integrative therapeutic intervention, examining its influence on physical self-concept, perceived pain reduction, disability, range of motion (ROM), muscular strength, and pelvic pain [3].

The compilation includes studies with diverse populations including women with chronic low back pain, individuals with various musculoskeletal disorders, and adolescents. By incorporating studies investigating the effects of SNPE on energy expenditure, exercise intensity, and specific pain-related factors, our understanding of SNPE's mechanisms and outcomes will be enriched [6].

The exploration extends to potential role of SNPE in conditions such as dysmenorrhea, premenstrual syndrome, and chronic knee pain, providing a holistic perspective on its versatility in enhancing overall well-being. This chapter aims to consolidate current research findings, shedding light on the intricate interplay between SNPE and various facets of musculoskeletal health. The diverse array of studies presented collectively contributes to the evolving narrative of SNPE as an innovative and effective approach to chronic pain management and therapy. This chapter would provide a comprehensive understanding of how SNPE may serve as a catalyst for change in physical function, posture, and pain perception.

2. Mechanism of SNPE

The SNPE is a specialized exercise method designed to independently correct misaligned spines and restore the natural posture of the human body through self-regulation. This targeted exercise focuses primarily on posture correction and draws inspiration from orthodontic principles.

2.1 Exercise components

SNPE utilizes specific belts, namely the posture correction belt and pelvic correction band, worn around the hips and legs, respectively.

The standard SNPE program consists of eight exercise units, including the 1st movement (Standing SNPE Signature Movements), 2nd movement (SNPE exercises performed while lying down), 3rd movement (SNPE exercises performed in the prone position), 4th movement (SNPE exercises performed while rolling), C-move (cervical movement), T-move (thoracic movement), L-move (lumbar movement), and

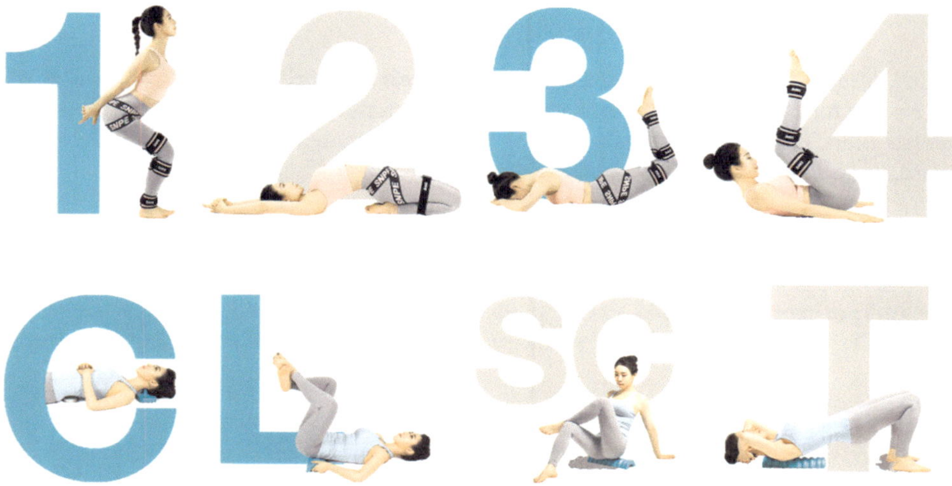

Figure 1.
Eight movements of SNPE. Adopted from https://snpelife.com/baseexercise/

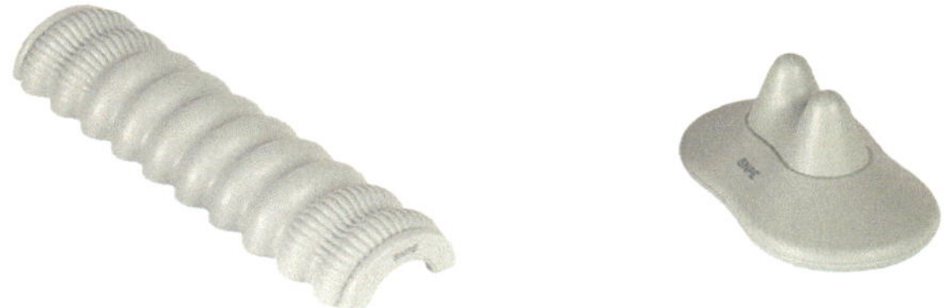

Figure 2.
(Left) Wave pillow and (Right) Danason (a neck massage tool). Adopted from http://snpeshop.com/

SC-move (sacrum-coccygeal movement) (**Figure 1**) [3, 5]. Integral to the exercise routine are complementary tools, such as the wave pillow, a basic tool (**Figure 2A**), Danason (a neck massage tool) (**Figure 2B**), and other tools such as the wave stick, that can be used for specific movements. These tools aid in alleviating spinal muscle tension and gradually correcting spinal deformities.

2.2 Orthodontic influence

SNPE incorporates sustained traction using prosthetics and elastic tools, akin to orthodontic practices. This approach, applied over time, allows for gradual dental correction. The potential application of such techniques to the SNPE belt in spinal correction exercises holds promise. The successful correction of rigid teeth, influenced by osteoblasts and osteocytes, suggests that this method may extend to correcting misaligned body postures. Consistent post-correction use of the SNPE belt, comparable to dental correction aids for preventing tooth misalignment, is considered crucial for avoiding relapse and maintaining preventive measures during body transformations. The distinctive features of SNPE spinal correction exercises can be summarized as the *3Us*:

2.2.1 United

Dr. Jungki Choi invented a comprehensive exercise method, integrating the study and research of various disciplines such as chiropractic care, yoga, Pilates, fitness, and diverse exercise therapies. This approach aims to alleviate and treat musculoskeletal disorders and pain.

2.2.2 Unique

A unique exercise method that applies the principles of orthodontics to the human body, utilizing the SNPE belt and spinal exercise tools as a novel therapeutic approach.

2.2.3 Useful (practical)

An effective exercise method for self-pain relief and proper posture correction, suitable for individuals of all ages and genders. This practical exercise can be performed in limited spaces, and it yields positive results in a short period.

3. Eight movements of SNPE

3.1 1st movements

3.1.1 Execution

- Wear SNPE posture correction belt and pelvic correction band.
- Stand straight, imagining there is a chair behind you.
- Sit deeply, expand the chest, arch the back, and shape hands like scissors.
- Shift weight to heels, raise toes, and lower the hips continuously.
- Key points: scissor-shaped hands, shift weight to the back, expand the chest.

3.1.2 Expected benefits

- Prevents neck disc and wrinkles by correcting the spine's shape.
- Prevents kyphosis, relieves shoulder pain by correcting posture.
- Prevents lower back pain and lumbar disc issues.
- Manage the postpartum body and correct pelvic alignment.
- Strengthens muscles, provides hip-lifting effects.
- Corrects bowlegs (O, X legs) (**Figure 3**).

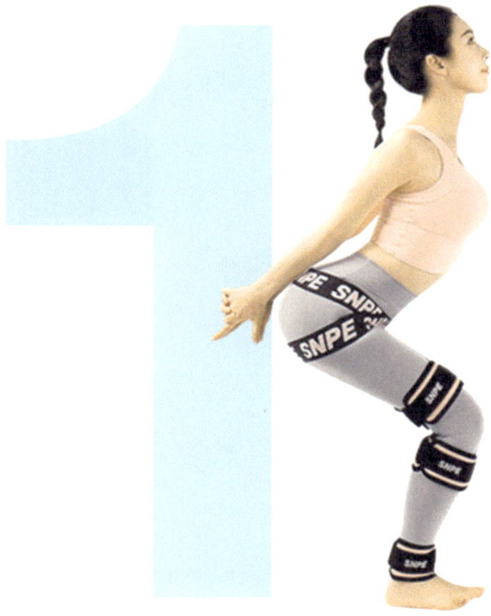

Figure 3.
1st movement of SNPE. Adopted from https://snpelife.com/baseexercise/

3.2 2nd movements

3.2.1 Execution

- Wear SNPE posture correction belt and pelvic correction band.
- Stretch calves using hands on the floor.
- Lie down, breathe, and engage abdominal and thigh muscles.
- Lower knees to the ground with exhalation and maintaining alignment.
- Keep shoulders, toes, and knees aligned for 1–3 minutes.
- Rise by tilting sideways after SNPE 2nd movement.

3.2.2 Expected benefits

- Corrects posture.
- Increases body temperature, aids digestion, prevents constipation, and alleviates menstrual pain.
- Relaxes tension in the transverse colon and enhances blood circulation.
- Relieves lower back pain and corrects pelvic alignment (**Figure 4**).

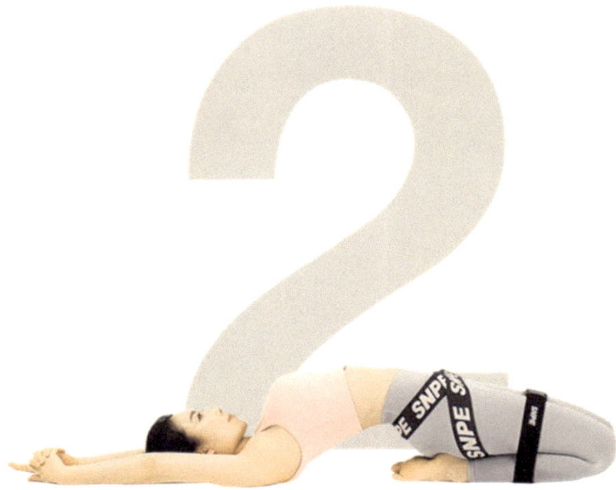

Figure 4.
2nd movement of SNPE. Adopted from https://snpelife.com/baseexercise/

3.3 3rd movements

3.3.1 Execution

- Lie down, tie legs with posture correction belt and pelvic correction band, and place hands under forehead.
- Lift legs, squeezing thighs, and buttocks.
- Maintain C-shaped waist curve for 10–20 seconds (5–10 sets).

3.3.2 Expected benefits

- Strengthens the waist, forms a C-shaped curve, and corrects pelvic balance.
- Raises body temperature.
- Corrects bowlegs (O, X legs) and knee misalignment.
- Strengthens waist and glutes muscles, and alleviates lower back pain.
- Corrects hip joints and pelvic alignment (**Figure** 5).

3.4 4th movements

3.4.1 Execution

- Roll backward from a seated position, raising toes over the head, then return to a bent position.

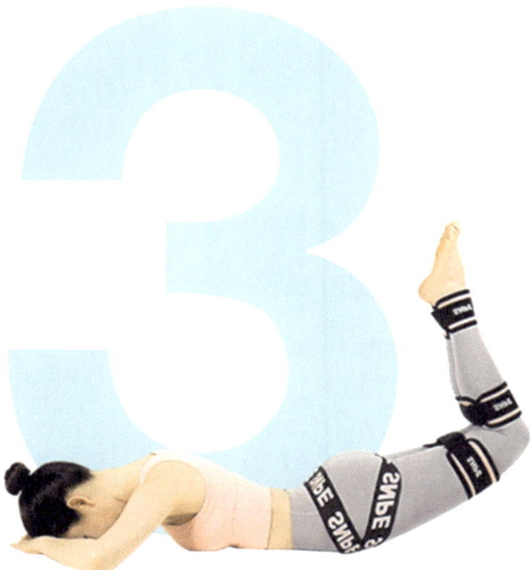

Figure 5.
3rd movement of SNPE. Adopted from https://snpelife.com/baseexercise/

3.4.2 Expected benefits

- Prevents and relieves pain in the neck, shoulders, back, lower back, pelvic pain, and muscle pain.
- Aids digestion, relieves constipation.
- Improves blood circulation.
- Corrects shoulder height, balances the back.
- Strengthens abdominal muscles (**Figure 6**).

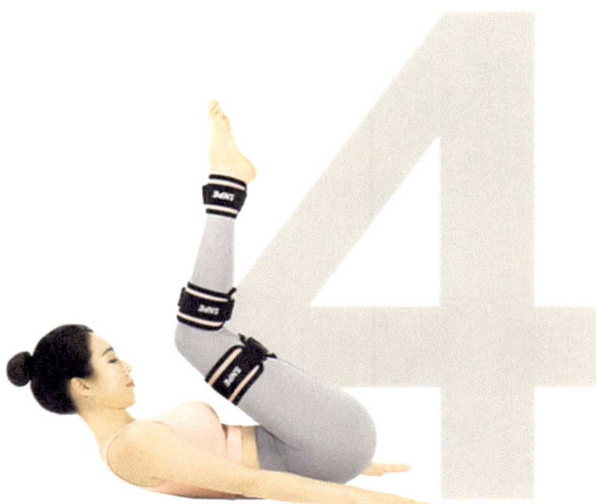

Figure 6.
4th movement of SNPE. Adopted from https://snpelife.com/baseexercise/

3.5 Cervical movement (C-move)

3.5.1 Execution

- Using wave pillow
  - Place the pillow under the neck or align with the hairline.
  - Move the head left and right, releasing tension.
  - Also, use the rounded part to massage the neck.
- Using Danason
  - Massage each vertebra by moving Danason along the hairline and neck boundary.
  - Use a towel under Danason for comfort.
  - Move Danason along each vertebra, applying pressure (1–3 minutes each).
  - Also, use a wooden hand tool.

3.5.2 Expected benefits

- Restore the straight neck (straightening C-curve) for prevention and relief.
- Prevent and alleviate neck disc, neck, and shoulder pain.
- Correct posture and prevent neck wrinkles (**Figure 7**).

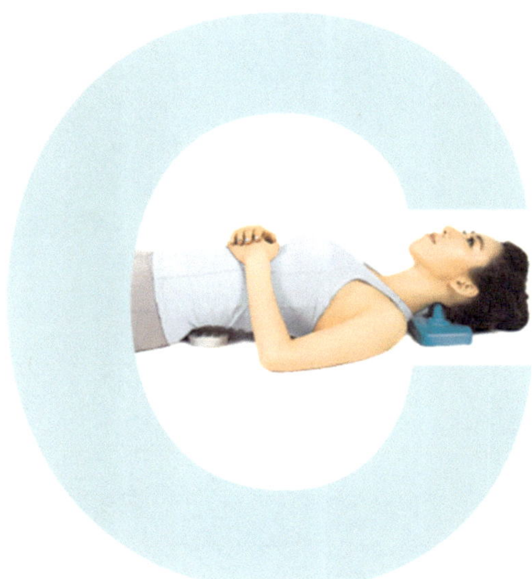

Figure 7.
C-movement of SNPE. Adopted from https://snpelife.com/baseexercise/

3.6 Thoracic movement (T-move)

3.6.1 Execution

- Using wave pillow.
    - Lie on the pillow vertically, knees up.
    - Raise and lower the pelvis while lifting the torso.
    - Repeat 30 times for 3–5 sets in various positions.
- Using Danason
    - Apply Danason under the hip and massage.
    - Move the body left and right while using Danason.

3.6.2 Expected benefits

- Prevent and correct the posture for a hunched back and rounded shoulders.
- Prevent rounding of the back, hunched shoulders, and associated symptoms.
- Assist in conditions such as frozen shoulder and correct rotator cuff abnormalities.
- Prevent and relieve forward head posture, straight neck, neck disc symptoms, and scoliosis (**Figure 8**).

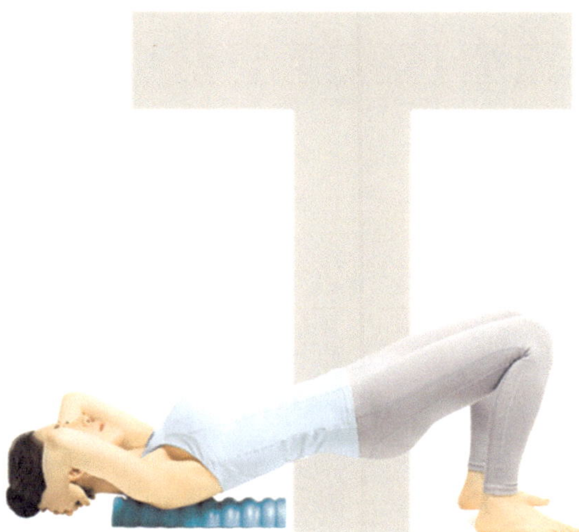

Figure 8.
T-movement of SNPE. Adopted from https://snpelife.com/baseexercise/

3.7 Lumbar movement (L-move)

3.7.1 Execution

- Using wave pillow
    - Place the pillow under the pelvis or waist.
    - Lift and lower legs to form a diamond shape.
    - Repeat 20–30 times for 3–5 sets.
    - Alternatively, use posture correction belt and pelvic correction band.

3.7.2 Expected benefits

- Correct the straightened lower back, forming a C-shaped curve.
- Alleviate lower back and pelvic pain, providing relief from lumbar disc issues.
- Relax stiff muscles in the lower back.
- Strengthen deep abdominal muscles, contributing to spinal stability.
- Reduce excess fat around the lower back and abdomen (**Figure 9**).

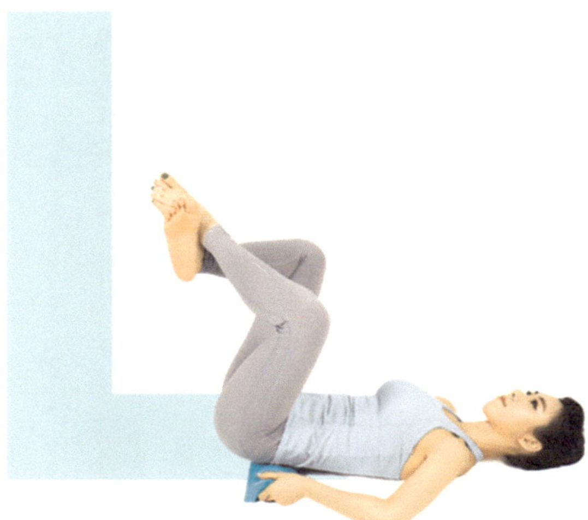

Figure 9.
L-movement of SNPE. Adopted from https://snpelife.com/baseexercise/

3.8 Sacrum-coccygeal movement (SC-move)

3.8.1 Execution

- Using wave pillow
  - Lie down with the pillow under the pelvis.
  - Move hips left and right to release muscles.
  - Tilt the pelvis for additional stretch.
- Using Danason
  - Press gently to release tension.
  - Consult a professional before starting a new exercise routine.

3.8.2 Expected benefits

- Correct pelvic alignment for improved posture.
- Alleviate pelvic pain and discomfort.
- Relax stiff muscles around the tailbone area.
- Relief lower back pain, tailbone pain, and hip joint pain (**Figure 10**).

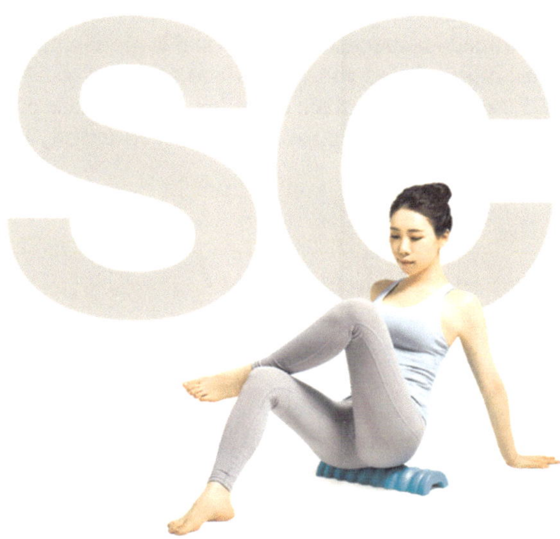

Figure 10.
SC-movement of SNPE. Adopted from https://snpelife.com/baseexercise/

4. Effects of SNPE on chronic pain

4.1 Effectiveness of SNPE in chronic pain management

The effectiveness of the SNPE program in managing chronic pain has been explored through various studies, highlighting its multifaceted impact on both physical and psychological dimensions. In an initial 12 weeks study [4, 5], participants undergoing the SNPE program reported significant improvements in muscle power, subjective health, flexibility, and a reduction in perceived pain. Significantly, a positive shift in physical self-concept was observed, highlighting the potential of SNPE as an intervention for chronic pain conditions [3].

4.2 Physical fitness and pain perception

A subsequent investigation examined the effects of SNPE on physical fitness, ROM, and pain perception among women with chronic musculoskeletal pain [6]. Positive outcomes were observed in flexibility, neck and shoulder ROM, waist flexion, hip rotation, and functional movement screen (FMS) outcomes. This suggests that SNPE not only enhances flexibility and ROM but also reduces pain perception in women with chronic musculoskeletal pain. Studies focusing on young women with chronic low back pain indicated significant improvements in the lumbar disorder index, lateral flexion, back strength, and pelvic pain release in the SNPE group [7]. This further supports SNPE's efficacy in various dimensions of health.

4.3 Moderating effects of SNPE self-efficacy

Another study explored the moderated mediating effect of SNPE self-efficacy on perceived pain through performance, revealing a significant correlation between higher self-efficacy and improved performance [8]. The perceived pain reduction effect was more pronounced in specific regions (waist, pelvis, hip, and knee) compared to shoulder pain, highlighting the specialized benefits of SNPE movements for different body areas. Examining affective complexity in female patients with chronic pain, a 12-week SNPE program led to pain and stress reduction, and increased life satisfaction [3].

5. Impact of SNPE on specific health issues

5.1 Correction of forward head posture (FHP) and neck pain

The study focused on young women with cervical discomfort and aimed to assess the impact of the 12 weeks SNPE program on FHP correction and neck pain relief [9]. The findings indicated a significant reduction in the distance between the centerline and ears, improvement in the craniovertebral angle (CVA), and decreased pain in trigger points, particularly in mastoid processes, vertebra prominens (C7), and upper trapezius (**Table 1**). These results suggest that SNPE is an effective exercise program for correcting FHP and alleviating neck pain [9].

Variables		Pre	Post	t	p
Posture	Ear_L (mm)	58.3 ± 22.1	41.5 ± 19.9	2.495	0.034
	Ear_R (mm)	52.0 ± 24.4	29.2 ± 21.5	2.861	0.019
	Acromion process_L (mm)	46.1 ± 26.3	35.6 ± 23.4	1.738	0.116
	Acromion process_R (mm)	52.7 ± 16.7	29.6 ± 28.3	3.067	0.013
	Glabella (mm)	9.9 ± 8.0	13.2 ± 7.6	−.991	0.348
	C7 (mm)	9.8 ± 7.8	5.9 ± 4.5	1.848	0.098
	Shoulder (mm)	6.6 ± 7.4	3.3 ± 6.3	1.383	0.200
	CVA (°)	46.1 ± 6.3	53.7 ± 8.1	−2.280	0.049
Pain	Mastoid process_L (score)	5.2 ± 1.7	1.0 ± 1.2	6.498	0.000
	Mastoid process_R (score)	5.1 ± 1.6	0.9 ± 0.9	10.088	0.000
	C7_L (score)	4.9 ± 2.0	1.5 ± 1.4	6.053	0.000
	C7_R (score)	4.6 ± 2.3	1.2 ± 1.1	4.841	0.001
	Upper trapezius_L (score)	5.1 ± 1.6	2.0 ± 1.2	5.670	0.000
	Upper trapezius_R (score)	5.3 ± 2.4	2.0 ± 0.9	4.337	0.002
	Supraspinatus_L (score)	5.3 ± 1.4	2.1 ± 1.4	6.000	0.000
	Supraspinatus_R (score)	5.5 ± 1.7	2.2 ± 2.0	5.706	0.000

Mean ± standard deviation.
CVA: craniovertebral angle.

Table 1.
Assessment of posture and cervical region pain.

5.2 Enhancing knee joint function and pain reduction

Examining women with chronic knee joint pain, a study revealed that the SNPE Lower Limb Conditioning Program effectively enhanced knee joint function, modified muscle tone, and reduced pain assessed by Western Ontario and McMaster Universities Osteoarthritis Index. The SNPE group demonstrated superiority over the control group, indicating its potential as an exercise for improving knee health by targeting joint function, pain reduction, and muscle tone modification [10].

5.3 Improvement in cervical and shoulder pain

A study focusing on women with chronic musculoskeletal pain investigated the impact of SNPE on cervical and shoulder pain as well as joint operating range. SNPE demonstrated significant improvements in cervical and shoulder pain, especially in cervical flexion and rotation (left) and shoulder mobility. This suggests that SNPE is beneficial for women with chronic musculoskeletal pain, indicating its effectiveness in improving specific regions [11].

5.4 Benefits for individuals with chronic spinal disorder

For individuals with chronic spinal diseases, SNPE showed notable benefits in pain reduction, muscle tone improvement, postural alignment, and skeletal structure changes. A customized SNPE program tailored to specific spinal diseases proved effective in enhancing muscle tone, correcting postural alignment, and contributing to pain relief in individuals with chronic spinal disorder [10, 11].

5.5 Posture correction and pain relief in young women with chronic neck pain

In women in their 20s and 30s experiencing chronic neck pain and forward head posture, SNPE demonstrated significant improvements in CVA, shoulder balance, overall body alignment, and pain relief. This suggests that the SNPE program is effective for correcting posture and alleviating neck pain in this specific demographic [9].

5.6 Pelvic misalignment and women's health

In another investigation, the effectiveness of SNPE in pelvic correction and menstrual symptom relief was evaluated in individuals with primary dysmenorrhea. The SNPE pelvic program resulted in decreased menstrual cramps, improved pelvic alignment, and positive changes in breast discomfort. These outcomes propose SNPE as an intervention for individuals with primary dysmenorrhea, showing potential benefits in pelvic alignment and symptom relief [12]. After 12 weeks of the SNPE program, the lumbar disorder index significantly decreased in the SNPEG group (pre: 7.6 ± 2.7 vs. post: 3.1 ± 2.7, $p < 0.001$). Lumbar flexion increased from 22.4 ± 2.7 to 26.8 ± 2.9 cm ($p < 0.05$), while extension decreased from 12.2 ± 1.0 to 10.9 ± 1.0 cm ($p < 0.05$). Left lateral flexion decreased from 46.8 ± 3.9 to 42.5 ± 2.7 cm, and back strength in the SNPEG group increased from 57.5 ± 13.4 to 72.6 ± 12.5 kg ($p < 0.001$) [13]. Furthermore, SNPE program decrease the pelvic pain (**Table 2**).

Pelvic misalignment in women is often associated with infertility, menstrual pain, and lower back discomfort [14, 15]. After childbirth, many women experience pain and discomfort attributed to misalignments [16]. Proper pelvic management is crucial for women's health. A warm body is conducive to women's health and fertility. Correcting misaligned pelvises contributes to body warmth, preventing issues arising from a cold body [17]. Pelvic misalignment impedes healthy childbirth, causing pain

Sites	Pre	Post	p
Sacrum left	4.6 ± 1.1	0.7 ± 0.9	≤0.05
Acrum right	3.0 ± 1.5	1.2 ± 1.3	
Iliopsoas left	6.5 ± 1.4	2.3 ± 1.5	
Iliopsoas right	5.8 ± 1.6	2.2 ± 1.6	
Lateral iliac crest left	4.7 ± 2.2	1.6 ± 1.9	
Lateral iliac crest right	5.7 ± 1.9	2.1 ± 1.6	
Adductor left	5.2 ± 2.5	2.5 ± 2.2	
Adductor right	6.3 ± 2.1	3.1 ± 2.4	
Gluteus maximus left	6.3 ± 2.2	1.8 ± 0.8	
Gluteus maximus right	6.4 ± 2.4	1.7 ± 0.8	

Mean ± standard deviation.

Table 2.
Pelvic pain assessment.

and complications during delivery [18]. Maintaining a properly aligned pelvis is essential for a pain-free and healthy childbirth experience. Pelvic misalignment due to childbirth can lead to various women's health issues. SNPE exercises have proven therapeutic effects for preventing and managing conditions such as lower back pain and menstrual pain [13–15].

6. Effects of SNPE on adolescents

6.1 The impact of poor posture on adolescents

Previous research indicates that poor posture in adolescents can lead to kyphosis and scoliosis, characterized by excessive backward bending of the thoracic and sacral vertebrae, and an exaggerated frontal curve in the lumbar region, respectively [19]. Good posture is closely linked to overall health, while poor posture is associated with various musculoskeletal conditions that develop gradually over time due to repeated strain [20, 21].

6.2 Factors contributing to musculoskeletal conditions

Factors such as the repeated use of specific body parts, uncomfortable postures, excessive strain, or overwork are known to cause minor damage to muscles, blood vessels, and nerves in joints, leading to chronic health issues in the musculoskeletal system accompanied by pain or dysesthesia [20, 21]. Musculoskeletal conditions evolve gradually due to prolonged exposure to adverse conditions, emphasizing the importance of implementing preventive measures.

6.3 Musculoskeletal health in adolescents

Adolescents, who often spend extended periods sitting at desks, may experience bodily imbalances due to insufficient physical activity, a lack of exercise, poor fitness, and postural instability, contributing to lumbar pain and even scoliosis [22]. In a study investigating the impact of rolling exercise with spinal stimulation on improving scoliosis in elementary school students, twelve 6th-grade students diagnosed with scoliosis were selected, with six in the experimental group and six in the control group. The rolling exercise, a component of the SNPE, was applied four times a week for 12 weeks. Cobb's angle was measured before and after the intervention to assess the exercise's effect [23]. The results revealed a positive impact of rolling exercise with spinal stimulation on thoracic Cobb's angle, indicating a significant improvement in the experimental group. This study highlights the potential benefits of incorporating simple and accessible exercises like rolling into school settings for the early detection and prevention of scoliosis among students.

The Cobb's angle is a crucial measurement in orthopedics to quantify the degree of curvature in the spine, particularly in the context of scoliosis. A larger Cobb's angle typically indicates a more substantial curvature of the spine [24]. In the pre-post comparison of the study investigating the effect of spine-stimulating rolling exercise on improving elementary school students' scoliosis, the experimental group showed a significant reduction in scoliosis. In contrast, the control group exhibited a worsening of scoliosis (**Table 3**). These findings emphasize the potential of simple exercises in school settings for early scoliosis detection and prevention.

Group	Pre	Post	t	P
Experiment	12.7 ± 6.9	7.2 ± 6.0	3.722	0.014
Control	11.5 ± 7.3	11.8 ± 8.1	−0.260	0.805
Mean ± standard deviation.				

Table 3.
Changes in thoracic Cobb's angle between pre and post SNPE program (°).

7. Effects of SNPE on fitness and functional movement

7.1 Pain perception and functional movement improvement

The investigation aimed to systematically evaluate the impact of a 12 weeks SNPE program on pain perception, functional movement, and fitness in women with chronic pain [3]. The exercise group demonstrated a significant reduction in pain perception, as assessed by the Short-Form McGill Pain Questionnaire (pre: 9.5 ± 7.2 vs. post: 3.5 ± 2.8, $p < 0.01$). FMS tests indicated improvements in various movements, with significant group differences observed. While both the exercise group and non-exercise group showed an increase in the FMS total score, the exercise group exhibited greater improvement in flexibility, measured by sit-and-reach and back extension, demonstrating that SNPE is a valuable exercise modality for reducing pain perception, enhancing functional movement, and improving flexibility in women with chronic pain [3].

7.2 Correlation between SNPE motion performance and musculoskeletal pain regions

Another study investigated the relationship between SNPE motion performance and musculoskeletal pain regions in adult women with chronic musculoskeletal pain. The evaluation focused on factors such as shoulder and pelvic balance, angles formed by specific body points, and shoulder position during 1st movement of SNPE. Significant relationships were found between motion performance and pressure pain thresholds in specific areas, providing insights into musculoskeletal pain regions associated with 1st movement of SNPE. This offers a basis for tailoring effective exercise programs to alleviate chronic musculoskeletal pain during SNPE exercise program [25].

7.3 Energy expenditure and exercise intensity evaluation

Furthermore, a study assessed the energy expenditure (EE) and exercise intensity (EI) of SNPE in women certified as skilled instructors, ranging from their 20s to 40s. Oxygen uptake (VO_2) and heart rates (HR) were measured during eight basic movements of SNPE. The 4th movement of SNPE demonstrated the highest EE and exhibited a statistically significant difference from the other 7 movements ($p < 0.05$), including the 1st, 2nd, 3rd, T, L, SC, and C-movement. The EI of SNPE movements was calculated based on the metabolic equivalent (MET) of task by employing the measured VO_2 (**Table 4**). The 4th movement of SNPE was categorized as vigorous intensity, while T, 1st, and L-movement were classified as moderate exercise intensity.

	VO_2 (ml/kg/min)	MET	HR (beats/min)
1st movement	13.7 ± 2.7	3.9 ± 0.8	123.5 ± 17.6
2nd movement	6.5 ± 1.5	1.9 ± 0.4	79.3 ± 13.6
3rd movement	10.3 ± 2.9	2.9 ± 0.8	107.2 ± 18.6
4th movement	21.5 ± 5.6	6.1 ± 1.6	121.8 ± 18.4
C-movement	5.3 ± 1.1	1.5 ± 0.3	75.6 ± 11.4
T-movement	15.7 ± 4.2	4.5 ± 1.2	107.7 ± 17.9
L-movement	11.6 ± 2.3	3.3 ± 0.7	98.9 ± 14.9
SC-movement	8.5 ± 2.5	2.4 ± 0.7	90.3 ± 12.2

Mean ± standard deviation.
VO_2; oxygen uptake, MET; metabolic equivalents, HR; heart rate.

Table 4.
Energy expenditure and exercise intensity of SNPE.

The other movements were determined as low EI, with the 3rd, SC, 2nd, and C-movement in order. However, HR exhibited a different order of EI, with the 1st, 4th, T, 3rd, L, SC, 2nd, and C-movement, respectively (**Table 4**). A significant difference was observed among the 1st, 4th, and the other 6 movements ($p < 0.05$) [13].

8. Limitations and future research

Numerous studies robustly affirm the versatility and effectiveness of SNPE in various dimensions of women's health. However, research on its application in men remains limited. Consequently, future studies are needed to explore the effectiveness of SNPE in correcting posture and alleviating pain in men. This chapter, therefore, lacks an analysis of potential gender differences in the utility and effectiveness of SNPE for these purposes. Future research should delve into SNPE's potential as a tailored and holistic exercise program applicable across diverse age groups and specific health conditions for both men and women.

9. Conclusions

In conclusion, the synthesis of diverse studies strongly supports the versatility and effectiveness of SNPE in various dimensions of women's health while it has not been extensively studied with men. SNPE's holistic approach, ranging from posture correction to targeted enhancements in joint function and pelvic health, positions it as a promising component of comprehensive pain treatment strategies.

The integration of these studies underlines SNPE's possibility as a tailored and holistic exercise program applicable across different age groups and specific health conditions. Notably, its positive impact on musculoskeletal health in adolescents highlights the importance of early detection and preventive measures through accessible exercises like rolling. This comprehensive research reinforces SNPE's utility and effectiveness in correcting posture, and alleviating pain. The integrated findings offer valuable insights for healthcare professionals, instructors, and individuals seeking structured exercise programs to manage and alleviate chronic pain. In essence, SNPE emerges as a multifaceted and effective intervention with broad applications in women's health and well-being, emphasizing its significant role in holistic health approaches.

Collectively, these findings substantiate SNPE as a multifaceted intervention that enhances physical aspects, including disability, ROM, and muscular strength. Moreover, SNPE has a positive impact on emotional well-being, affective complexity, and self-regulation. SNPE distinguishes itself as a personalized and effective approach to pain management, delivering specialized benefits for different body regions.

Conflict of interest

The authors declare no conflict of interest.

Author details

Yongsuk Seo and Dae Taek Lee*
Kookmin University, Seoul, Republic of Korea

*Address all correspondence to: dtlee@kookmin.ac.kr

References

[1] Busk H, Ahler J, Bricca A, Holm MP, Poulsen DV, Skou ST, et al. Exercise-based rehabilitation in and with nature: A scoping review mapping available interventions. Annals of Medicine. 2023; **55**(2):2267083

[2] Stoewen DL. Dimensions of wellness: Change your habits, change your life. The Canadian Veterinary Journal. 2017; **58**(8):861-862

[3] Choi J, Yoon J, Shin M. Effects of pain reduction by self-natural posture exercise on affective complexity in women: The moderating effect of self-regulation. Frontiers in Psychology. 2020;**11**:1317

[4] Mills SEE, Nicolson KP, Smith BH. Chronic pain: A review of its epidemiology and associated factors in population-based studies. British Journal of Anaesthesia. 2019;**123**(2): e273-ee83

[5] Yoon J, Choi J, Shin M. Self-natural posture exercise and chronic pain reduction. SBP Journal. 2019;**47**(11): 1-11

[6] Kim S. Determination of Energy Expenditure and Exercise Intensity of SNPE [MS Thesis]. Kookmin University; 2021

[7] Lee H, Yun S, Lee Y, Lee DT, Yoon J, Kyeong J. Effects of the SNPE (self natural posture exercise) program for disability, range of motion, muscular strength, and pelvic pain in patients with chronic low back pain. Journal of the Korean Society for Wellness. 2022;**17**(1): 245-252

[8] Choi J, Yoon J, Shin M. Effect of SNPE self-efficacy on the reduction of chronic pain mediated by performance depending on regional pain. KSSO. 2019; **17**(4):661-671

[9] Lee H, Yoon J, Choi J, Yun S, Hwang JG, Lee Y, et al. Effects of SNPE program on postural correction and neck pain relief in women with forward head posture. Journal of the Korean Society for Wellness. 2020;**15**:565-573

[10] Lee H, Yoon J, Lee DT. Effect of SNPE program on knee joint function, pain, and muscle tone in women with chronic knee pain: 1270. Medicine & Science in Sports & Exercise. 2022;**54** (9S):314-315

[11] Kim S, Lee H, Lee H, Yoon J, Lee DT. Effects of SNPE shoulder conditioning program on shoulder pain and function in women with chronic shoulder pain: 2819. Medicine & Science in Sports & Exercise. 2023;**55**(9S):961-962

[12] Kim H, Lee H, Yoon J, Lee DT. Effects of SNPE program on pelvic alignment, dysmenorrhea, and premenstrual syndrome: 2832. Medicine & Science in Sports & Exercise. 2023;**55**(9S):966-967

[13] Lee H, Yoon J, Choi J, Kyeong J, Yun S, Lee Y, et al. Effectiveness of SNPE on disability, range of motion, muscular strength, and pelvic pain in women with chronic low back pain: 1125 Board #251 May 27 2:30 PM - 4:00 PM. Medicine & Science in Sports & Exercise. 2020;**52**:293

[14] Walicka-Cupryś K, Pelc AR, Pasierb M, Płonka S, Pal A, Rosowska N. Effect of lumbar spine mobility and postural alignment on menstrual pain in young women. International Journal of Environmental Research and Public Health. 2023;**20**(15):6458

[15] Minicozzi SJ, Russell BS, Ray KJ, Struebing AY, Owens EF Jr. Low back pain response to pelvic tilt position: An observational study of chiropractic patients. Journal of Chiropractic Medicine. 2016;**15**(1):27-34

[16] Katonis P, Kampouroglou A, Aggelopoulos A, Kakavelakis K, Lykoudis S, Makrigiannakis A, et al. Pregnancy-related low back pain. Hippokratia. 2011;**15**(3):205-210

[17] Sharma R, Biedenharn KR, Fedor JM, Agarwal A. Lifestyle factors and reproductive health: Taking control of your fertility. Reproductive Biology and Endocrinology. 2013;**11**:66

[18] Morino S, Ishihara M, Umezaki F, Hatanaka H, Yamashita M, Aoyama T. Pelvic alignment changes during the perinatal period. PLoS One. 2019;**14**(10): e0223776

[19] Geldhof E, De Clercq D, De Bourdeaudhuij I, Cardon G. Classroom postures of 8-12 year old children. Ergonomics. 2007;**50**(10): 1571-1581

[20] Odebiyi DO, Okafor UAC. Musculoskeletal disorders, workplace ergonomics and injury prevention. In: Orhan K, editor. Ergonomics. Rijeka: IntechOpen; 2023. p. Ch. 2

[21] Shumway NK, Cole E, Fernandez KH. Neurocutaneous disease: Neurocutaneous dysesthesias. Journal of the American Academy of Dermatology. 2016;**74**(2):215-228

[22] Bull FC, Al-Ansari SS, Biddle S, Borodulin K, Buman MP, Cardon G, et al. World Health Organization 2020 guidelines on physical activity and sedentary behaviour. British Journal of Sports Medicine. 2020;**54**(24): 1451-1462

[23] Kim MJ. The Effect of Rolling Exercise with Spinal Stimulation on Improvement of Scoliosis in Elementary School Students with Focus on the SNPE 4th Exercise [MS Thesis]. Seoul National University of Education; 2022

[24] Horng MH, Kuok CP, Fu MJ, Lin CJ, Sun YN. Cobb angle measurement of spine from X-Ray images using convolutional neural network. Computational and Mathematical Methods in Medicine. 2019;**2019**:6357171

[25] Lee H, Yoon J, Kyeong J, Jeon J, Kim H, Kim S, et al. Effects of SNPE program on factors of pain in patient with dorsopathies: 1367. Medicine & Science in Sports & Exercise. 2021; **53**:449

Chapter 8

Using Burst Modality Medium Frequency Alternating (Russian and Aussie) Currents with Isokinetic Training

Musa Çankaya and İlkim Çıtak Karakaya

Abstract

Isokinetic exercises are a type of exercise that can be performed both concentrically and eccentrically at various angular velocities while applying resistance to the muscles at each point of the range of motion. These exercises are known to have many benefits compared to other exercises. Electrotherapy modalities are a popular treatment used by physiotherapists for a variety of purposes, such as muscle strengthening, endurance, spasticity management, pain control, circulation enhancement, and edema control. Kilohertz-frequency alternating currents were introduced in the pioneering work of Kots as a new form of neuromuscular electrical stimulation that was believed to solve some of the limitations of conventional electrical stimulation. Russian current is a medium-frequency alternating current that is delivered in bursts, with the carrier frequency ranging from 1000 to 10,000 Hz and any burst frequency being acceptable. Aussie currents are utilized in clinics at 1000 Hz, modulated in 50 Hz intervals with a pulse duration of 2 msec. Medium-frequency currents, particularly Russian and Aussie currents in isokinetic training, provide muscle strength contraction and endurance, increased blood circulation, and specific physiological effects. Considering the person's health status, existing injuries, or other health problems, Russian and Aussie currents can be used effectively in isokinetic training at appropriate levels under the guidance of a physician and physiotherapist.

Keywords: isokinetic contraction, strength dynamometer, electrostimulation, Russian current, physiotherapy

1. Introduction

1.1 Isokinetic training

Isokinetic Exercises (IE) was first described by James Perrine in the 1960s. During IE, force is generated at a constant speed throughout the range of motion of the joint, and maximum force is generated in the muscle at every angle of the movement during contraction [1]. IE is a continuous constant speed training module. The speed of movement is constant except for acceleration at the beginning and deceleration at the end [2]. Isokinetic force is the highest torque (rotational moment) value developed during contraction at a given speed. IE can be performed concentrically and eccentrically at different angular velocities applies resistance to the muscles at each point of the range of motion and is well known to have many advantages over other exercises [3]. IE provides better strengthening compared to isometric and isotonic exercises because it allows eccentric contractions that can provide more strength and endurance increase in the muscle throughout the entire range of motion [4]. IE provides usable and reliable data at low, medium, and high speed for assessment and rehabilitation programs. IE can be used as a personalized muscle-strengthening technique. It offers a gradual and safe exercise program with objective measurement of muscle strength increase. While exercise offers great selectivity in movement, it produces faster strength gains and less muscle sensitivity than isotonic training. In addition, heart rate and blood pressure increases are lower than isometric exercise [5]. It has been reported that IE provides many benefits such as muscle strength, muscle endurance, and enzyme activities [6].

The isokinetic training used for the knee joint eliminates the bioarticular function of the hamstrings. The position of extended hip flexion from the trunk and increased hip flexion from the corresponding femur make the typical hamstring tension more functional as a mechanism [7]. Isokinetic training is the only safe way to load dynamically contracted muscles to maximum capacity throughout their entire range in a continuous movement using functional positions or isolated in correct biomechanical positions. Isokinetic contraction engages more muscle fibers than any other exercise method (**Figure 1**) [8]. The mechanism of isokinetic training has been explained by improvement in muscle performance, speed-specific adaptation of motor units within the muscle, and speed-specific adaptation in the nervous system. However, differences in the direction of the transfer effect can be explained by differences in sample size, muscle fiber distribution, and training duration and intensity [9]. Vidmar et al. studied, that the peak torque of the traditional training group before treatment was concentric 176.6, eccentric 109.1, and after treatment peak torque was concentric 205.7 and eccentric 128.8. In the isokinetic training group, pre-treatment peak torque concentric 165.1, eccentric 97.7, post-treatment peak torque concentric 206.0, and eccentric 162.1 [10]. Isokinetic eccentric training appears to have a greater effect on quadriceps muscle mass and muscle mass than traditional eccentric training [10].

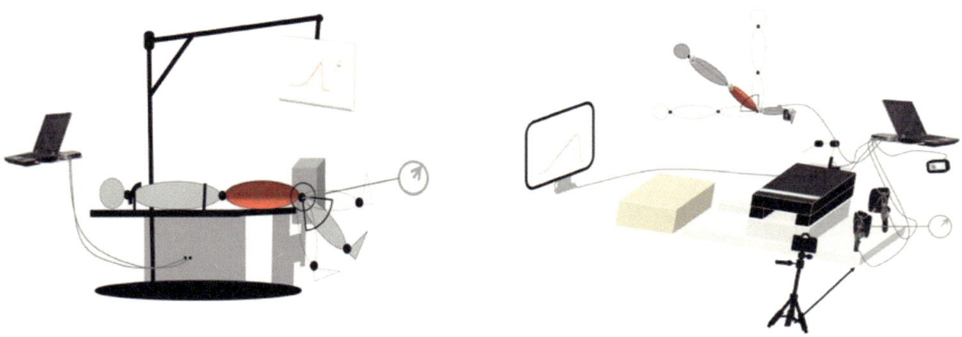

Figure 1.
Isokinetic dynamometer mechanism and effects of isokinetic training.

Petrucci et al. [11] review reported that in two studies included in their systematic review, isokinetic training produced significant differences ($p < 0.05$) in terms of increased muscle mass compared to the isotonic group. Tsaklis et al. [12] showed in their study that pre-post differences in muscle mass were higher in the isokinetic group, but no significant results were obtained. Therefore, it is recommended in the study that isokinetic training should be preferentially used instead of traditional isotonic to improve postoperative muscle mass. Sekir et al. [13] study, the peak torque concentric evertor of the ankle joint on the injured side before exercise was 15.54, the inverter 14.79, and the peak torque concentric evertor after exercise was 17.21, the invertor 16.50. The peak torque concentric evertor of the intact side ankle joint before exercise was 16.96, inverter 17.46, and the peak torque concentric evertor after exercise was 17.38, inverter 16.92. After the treatment, it is observed that the muscle strength between the injured and intact sides is similar. It is stated that the functional capacity of the injured ankle reaches the same level as the healthy ankle.

1.2 Isokinetic dynamometers

Assessing muscular strength using an isokinetic device is now widely used for various purposes, including rehabilitation of muscular and connective tissue injuries [14]. After quantitative measurement of muscle strength, the range of motion in which the muscle is weak can be determined. An appropriate exercise program can then be designed for the patient [15]. In addition, it allows kinematic analysis of movement in parameters such as determining agonist/antagonist muscle strength ratios, comparing both sides in limb segments, and measuring muscle work capacity and endurance. Isokinetic testing measures muscles or muscle groups in isolation. In cases where weak muscles are compensated by strong muscles, functional capacity is fully assessed. Measurements can be repeated and speed of movement can be determined (**Figure 2**) [4].

The isokinetic dynamometer is recognized as a valid method of assessing muscle strength and is often used as a reference standard for other strength assessments [16, 17]. An isokinetic dynamometer allows the assessment of muscle function with an appropriate resistance at a constant angular velocity, allowing maximum force

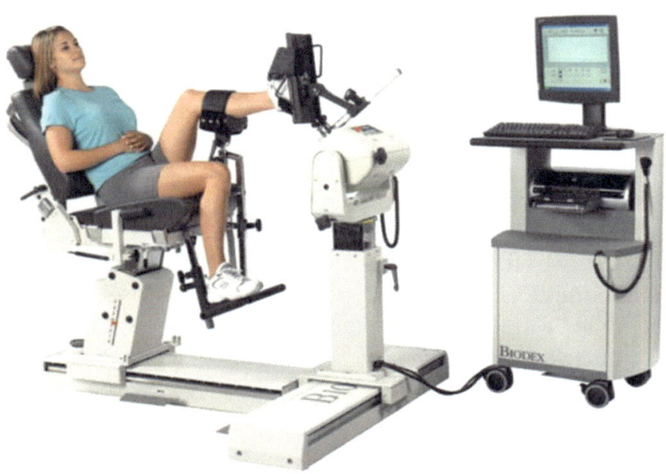

Figure 2.
Isokinetic dynamometer.

production through a prescribed range of motion. In clinical practice, isokinetic dynamometers are often preferred to monitor progress during rehabilitation [17].

Isokinetic dynamometers can assess muscle strength in both the concentric and eccentric phases of movement. Eccentric muscle activity is superior to concentric contraction in many ways. Approximately 40–60% more strength gain can be achieved with eccentric muscle contraction. It also has a beneficial effect on inflammation by altering blood flow [3].

In isokinetic dynamometry, the speed of the moving segment cannot exceed a predetermined speed, no matter how much force is applied. It is therefore safe to use in the rehabilitation of patients with muscle and ligament injuries. In addition, these machines provide an objective measure of muscle strength, power, and endurance. As a result, they are increasingly being used to assess muscle performance. Isokinetic equipment is now used for strength training and rehabilitation, as well as to determine muscle balance and strength [17].

Current isokinetic dynamometer systems allow assessment in both concentric and eccentric exercise modes. The dynamometer shows the value of the developing force moment at each moment. In addition, the muscle is maximally loaded at a predetermined constant speed and during dynamic movement [18]. The most important data recorded by the isokinetic dynamometer is the battery torque or maximum force moment, which indicates the highest force value recorded during the test. Another variable provided by the isokinetic dynamometer is "work", which is the product of force moment and angular distance.

Isokinetic dynamometers are mostly used to analyze peak torque data [19]. Isokinetic dynamometers are used to perform exercises at maximum intensity and constant angular velocity throughout the range of motion. This allows the exercise to be performed at the individual's maximum strength level at each joint angle and minimizes the risk of overloading the patient's tolerance. Isokinetic exercise is included in rehabilitation programs to optimize muscular strength, particularly in the treatment of elite athletes [10].

Studies have reported increases in maximal strength and endurance performance with IE [20]. Isokinetic dynamometers are the gold standard for assessing muscle strength, allowing us to determine the agonist/antagonist ratio through different angular velocities. It is also considered an effective tool for improving muscle function. Isokinetic dynamometry was introduced as a trade name in the late 1960s with the first Cybex I machine. Since then, much research has been conducted in the field of rehabilitation and sports performance, with the knee joint being the most studied and the hip to a lesser extent [20].

Isokinetic dynamometers are widely used in both clinical and research settings. In the literature, most studies using isokinetic dynamometers have focused on knee flexors and extensors, with less attention paid to the hip joint (14). In a systematic review, isokinetic knee flexion and extension force measurements using a wide range of angular velocities were reported to provide moderate to good reliability [14]. Although the reliability of isokinetic assessments is influenced by factors such as the position of the person, movement speed, muscle contraction, and pelvic stability, according to the results of the meta-analysis, they have produced measurements with higher reliability [20].

1.3 Isokinetic strength measurement

Determination of angular velocities There is a wide range of angular velocities used to test the quadriceps and hamstring group muscles. In 1989, Borges preferred a very low speed of 12°/sec, while at the other end of the spectrum. Ghena et al. [6] tested subjects at speeds up to 500°/sec. For the knee joint, velocities above 180°/sec are defined as high velocities [6, 21]. The gain increase at high angular velocities and whether it provides meaningful data is controversial. In the isokinetic dynamometer, as the angular speed increases, the maximum torque decreases. Again, some studies reported that very little muscle force change was detected at speeds above 300°/sec in the knee, and the maximum change was obtained between 30 and 120°/sec [22]. In conclusion, in light of the studies in the literature, the angular velocities between 60 and 180°/sec are the ones that are comfortable for the patient during isokinetic testing and allow for obtaining adequate and reliable data in terms of muscle performance [23].

The isokinetic dynamometer is the gold standard for measuring peak torque, work, and force as a function of angular velocity, as well as the agonist/antagonist muscle force ratio. Peak torque is a good indicator of maximum muscle tension, and strength tests are performed at low speeds (30–60°/s), while endurance and total work tests are performed at high speeds (180–300°/s). Total work is the sum of all the work performed in one set. Total work is used to measure endurance in isokinetic testing [24].

When the literature is examined, it is stated that electrotherapy methods should be combined with isokinetic training and the use of electrophysical agents [25–27]. Isokinetic training can be used in many diseases. Isokinetic training is as effective as traditional isotonic training in regaining strength and balance between hamstrings and quadriceps and results in better adaptation in muscle mass. As a result, isokinetic training is included as one of the main strength restoration strategies after knee surgery rehabilitation, especially in the early and intermediate stages when strength restoration is one of the main goals [28]. In a study, it was reported that Russian Current and High Voltage Pulsed Current (HVPC), which can be added to isokinetic strengthening exercises, have the same effect on muscle strength and endurance. It has been shown that both currents can be used to increase muscle endurance. Therefore, physiotherapists can plan a program that includes electrotherapy methods and isokinetic training, especially if they want to improve muscular endurance [29].

2. Limitations

When systematic reviews and meta-analyses were examined, it was determined that although isokinetic strength assessment is the gold standard, its general role is limited. However, best evidence syntheses, coupled with considerations of costs and the specialized training required to perform isokinetic strength testing, make this test difficult to use as a screening tool. For measurement, the patient who is being measured must be well informed and the professional who will make the measurement must be able to use the isokinetic dynamometer well. In addition, although measurements can be made in every region thanks to the apparatus in the device, it is difficult and time-consuming to use. Since the patient's motivation to perform the movement comes into play during the measurement, there may be problems with measurement consistency.

3. Electrotherapy methods

Electrotherapy modalities are a popular treatment used by physiotherapists for a variety of purposes including muscle strengthening, endurance, spasticity management, pain control, circulation enhancement, and edema control [30]. Medium-frequency currents are typically 2 kHz or 4 kHz modulated alternating currents [31]. The kilohertz-frequency alternating current waveform is a sinusoidal, triangular, or rectangular-shaped biphasic current. They are transmitted continuously or in bursts. It is defined as a current with a carrier frequency of 1.0–10.0 kHz and is usually modulated with a low frequency (1–120 Hz) because continuous alternating current rapidly causes neuromuscular fatigue due to high frequency [32]. Medium-frequency currents have a carrier frequency (excitation without pauses in the pulse) and a modulation frequency (the number of times the current modulates or changes in one second). The currents must have an excitation and rest period to resemble a voluntary contraction. These values are adjustable, the unit is sec. The greater the pulse duration and frequency, the greater the contraction. Increasing these parameters will increase discomfort and fatigue [33]. In the classical literature, mid-frequency neuromuscular electrical stimulation includes Russian currents and interference currents [31]. Neo-Russian currents, which differ from traditional Russian currents in various technical aspects, are included in this list. Aussie currents, which have recently been more widely used and attracted attention, are among these currents [34].

Kilohertz alternating current was proposed in the pioneering work of Kots as a new type of neuromuscular electrical stimulation (NMES) that would address some of the limitations of conventional electrical stimulation. There is evidence to suggest that kilohertz alternating current (hereafter referred to as Russian current) increases maximal voluntary isometric contraction by up to 40%. It has been reported that kilohertz alternating current produces suprathreshold stimuli with bursts long enough to generate multiple nerve fiber action potentials, producing smaller perturbations per burst and more force than conventional NMES [32].

4. Russian current

Russian Current (RA) was developed by Yakov Kots in the late 1970s to strengthen the quadriceps of Russian Olympic athletes. RA was developed as an electrical muscle stimulation to increase strength gains [35]. The key feature of RA is its ability to produce a large muscle contraction with repetitive external loading [36].

RA is a medium frequency alternating current transmitted in bursts where the carrier frequency is between 1000 and 10,000 Hz and any burst frequency can be used. The RA protocol medium frequency alternating carrier frequency is 2500 Hz. It is a 50-burst modulated current per second during 10 msec rest and 10 msec stimulation. The theoretical basis for its use is that the skin provides less resistance to the high carrier frequency of 2500 Hz and the RA stimulates almost all motor units of the muscle to contract simultaneously leading to greater muscle hypertrophy. This allows less electrical energy to be dissipated peripherally and more electrical energy to penetrate the muscle and stimulate more fiber release [36]. RA has gained popularity among athletes with Kots' reports of strength gain, 2500 Hz frequencies, 50 Hz bursts, and 50% duty cycle [37]. The RA protocol used in the clinic uses a medium frequency alternating current carrier frequency of 2500 Hz and a burst frequency of 50 bursts/second [38]. Akınoğlu et al. [39] evaluated isokinetic training with Russian current (RC) and high voltage pulsed current (HVPC) modality before and after treatment with isokinetic tests. Knee extension peak torque values 180°/sec before treatment RC is 161.60, HVPC is 157.50, after treatment, RC is 185.10, HVPC is 178.45. Quadriceps muscle 180°/sec muscular endurance before treatment RC is 72.02, HVPC is 69.88, post-treatment RC is 79.75, HVPC is 73.43. After the treatment, peak torque and muscular endurance increased.

5. Aussie current

Aussie Current (AC) is a 1 kHz or 4 kHz low-frequency alternating current that can modulate the duty cycle by 20%. Aussie currents are used in the clinic at 1000 Hz, modulated in 50 Hz ranges with a pulse duration of 2 msec [37]. AA can vary between 1 and 180 mA according to the sensitivity of the patient. A burst modulation frequency between 100 and 120 Hz is used for pain. It is a current that is rarely described in the physiotherapy literature, but its use as a way of increasing blood flow to the muscles as well as reducing pain has attracted attention [40].

Cittadino et al. [37] compared RA and AC applied to the hand in their study. Muscle strength and thickness of hand muscles were examined. In both evaluations, the average muscle thickness and effect sizes of the groups were determined as RA group 1.3 and AC group 1.7 in the first evaluation of the superficial flexors, and RA group 1.6 and AC group 1.7 after the treatment. The deep flexors were 1.7 in the RA group and 2.3 in the AC group at the first evaluation, and after treatment, they were 2.0 in the RA group and 2.3 in the AC group. No significant difference was found between the groups after treatment.

Dantas et al. [40] study, the authors compared RC and AC, as well as two other low-frequency currents with a phase duration of 200 or 500 us. The results showed that the maximum voluntary contraction torque applied in isolation was AC: 76.9%; and RC: 70.1%. Average torque AC: 92.1 percent; RC: 92.3 percent. There is no significant difference between the average torques. All currents are stated to produce similar levels of discomfort. Similar results were obtained by Ward et al., but both AC and RC have lower disturbance levels compared to low-frequency currents [41]. Medeiros et al. [42] also compared 1 and 4 kHz with two low-frequency currents with similar phase durations and observed that they presented similar levels of induced torque and discomfort. This form of treatment is relatively new and there are few studies examining its clinical effects. Current studies indicate that a new current, known as AC, can produce higher torque [43]. AC has a variety of therapeutic effects for individuals, including greater comfort, motor and sensory stimulation, and the capacity to produce greater muscle power torque [34]. Rodrigo et al. [43] reported that neuromuscular electrical stimulation provided by AC increased quadriceps muscle endurance in sedentary individuals and modulation with a 4 msec burst showed better effects. Dantas et al. [40] reported that Aussie current and low-frequency current were superior to Russian current for stimulating isometric knee extension torque.

	Frequency (Hz)	Bursts (Hz)	Duty cycle (%)	Rest and stimulation
Russian current	2500	50	50	10 msec rest and 10 msec stimulation
Aussie current	1000	50	20	2 msec stimulation

Table 1.
Russian and Aussie current application parameters.

This information is thought to be important in making decisions regarding physiotherapy protocols for muscle strengthening [40]. AC has been reported to have better torque and force gains compared to other electrotherapy modulations. It causes less discomfort to the patient and shows higher individual tolerance (**Table 1**).

6. Burst modality medium frequency currents (Russian and Aussie currents) in isokinetic training

The movement of the extremities in isokinetic training is performed at a predetermined speed during the joint movement process, except for the instantaneous acceleration at the beginning and deceleration at the end of the movement, known as isokinetic strength training [44]. Isokinetic training has been reported in research to be more effective than traditional isotonic training in restoring strength and balance between hamstrings and quadriceps. It causes better adaptations in muscle mass. Isokinetic training is among the most important methods in the development of functional mobility [28]. Vidmar et al. reported that isokinetic muscle strength training had a greater effect on muscle mass and strength of quadriceps femoris in recreational athletes after anterior cruciate ligament reconstruction than traditional training [10]. Some studies show that isokinetic training not only improves pain and dysfunction but also has a beneficial effect on the level of inflammatory biomarkers for college football players with traumatic osteoarthritis after anterior cruciate ligament injury and knee anterior cruciate ligament reconstruction revision patients [45, 46].

Isokinetic exercises are an exercise method used to increase muscle strength and improve performance.

These exercises are usually based on working with resistance and aim to work the muscles at maximum strength. The use of medium-frequency currents, especially Russian and Aussie currents in isokinetic training, provides muscle strength contraction and endurance, and increased blood circulation, along with certain physiological effects [29, 37]. Considering the health status of the person, existing injuries, or other health problems, Russ and Aussie currents can be used effectively in isokinetic training at appropriate levels under the guidance of a physician and physiotherapist.

From the literature review, it is seen that kHz current is a clinical alternative to add torque and muscle hypertrophy in healthy individuals. Although the force increase in the muscles occurs with other currents, it is seen that this increase occurs the most with the Russian current [47]. Since Aussie currents and Russian currents are similar in parameters, it is thought to be effective with isokinetic training. Although Aussie currents are few in the literature, no studies are used with isokinetic training. More research needs to be done on this subject. In addition, there are differences between the studies in terms of the parameters of the mid-frequency currents used. Therefore, more research can be done on current parameters.

7. Conclusions

Isokinetic training is a treatment modality used in the literature in the treatment of many diseases and is the best method for muscle strengthening. Burst modality medium frequency alternating currents are used in the literature. However, there are few studies conducted with isokinetic training. Although studies are showing that the Russian Current is effective among these currents, few studies are showing the effectiveness of Aussie currents. Since Aussie currents are more conformable than Russian currents, they can be used more frequently on patients.

Acknowledgements

We would like to inform you that this study is a part of the PhD Thesis by the first author, which was supported by the Muğla Sıtkı Koçman University Scientific Research Projects Coordination Office (Project Grant Number 21/125/01/3/4, and the title "Comparison of the Efficacy of Russian and Aussie Currents with Isokinetic Exercise in Individuals with Patellofemoral Pain Syndrome: Randomized Controlled Study").

Conflict of interest

There is no conflict of interest for any of the authors.

Author details

Musa Çankaya[1*] and İlkim Çıtak Karakaya[2]

1 Department of Physiotherapy and Rehabilitation, Necmettin Erbakan University, Konya, Turkey

2 Department of Physiotherapy and Rehabilitation, Mugla Sıtkı Kocman University, Mugla, Turkey

*Address all correspondence to: musa-cankaya@hotmail.com

References

[1] Tugba K, Kaya E, Akinoglu B, Karaaslan Y, Un Yildirim N, Hasanoglu A. The effects of isokinetic strength training on strength at different angular velocities: A pilot study. Turkish. Journal of Sports Medicine. 2017;**52**(3):77-83. DOI: 10.5152/tjsm.2017.073

[2] McAlindon TE, Bannuru RR, Sullivan MC, Arden NK, Berenbaum F, et al. OARSI guidelines for the non-surgical management of knee osteoarthritis. Osteoarthritis and Cartilage. 2014, 2014;**22**(3):363-388. DOI: 10.1016/j.joca.2014.01.003

[3] Toprak EK, Ünver F, Kılıç Erkek Ö, Korkmaz H, Oymak B, Özdemir Y, et al. Aktif erkek bireylerde tek seans uygulanan izokinetik egzersizin DNA hasarı üzerine etkilerinin incelenmesi. Pamukkale Medical Journal. 2019;**12**(1):33-40. DOI: 10.31362/patd.46351

[4] Gökçen N, Benlidayı İC, Başaran S. Isokinetic test and exercises in knee osteoarthritis. Archives Medical Review Journal. 2015;**24**(2):228-238

[5] Coudeyre E, Jegu AG, Giustanini M, Marrel JP, Edouard P, Pereira B. Isokinetic muscle strengthening for knee osteoarthritis: A systematic review of randomized controlled trials with meta-analysis. Annals of Physical and Rehabilitation Medicine. 2016;**59**(3):207-215. DOI: 10.1016/j.rehab.2016.01.013

[6] Ghena DR, Kurth AL, Thomas M, Mayhew J. Torque characteristics of the quadriceps and hamstring muscles during concentric and eccentric loading. The Journal of Orthopaedic and Sports Physical Therapy. 1991;**14**(4):149-154. DOI: 10.2519/jospt.1991.14.4.149

[7] Brown R, Greig M. The influence of isokinetic dynamometer configuration on eccentric hamstring strength metrics: Implications for testing and training. Research in Sports Medicine. 2024;**32**(1):98-106

[8] Davies GJ, Ellenbecker TS, Andrews JR, Harrelson GL, Wilk KE. Application of isokinetics in testing and rehabilitation. Physical Rehabilitation of the Injured Athlete. 2004

[9] DA BVB. Isokinetic dynamometry applications and limitations. Sports Medicine. 1989;**8**(2):101-116

[10] Vidmar MF, Baroni BM, Michelin AF, Mezzomo M, Lugokenski R, Pimentel GL, et al. Isokinetic eccentric training is more effective than constant load eccentric training for quadriceps rehabilitation following anterior cruciate ligament reconstruction: A randomized controlled trial. Brazilian Journal of Physical Therapy. 2020;**24**(5):424-432. DOI: 10.1016/j.bjpt.2019.07.003

[11] Petrucci A, Guglielmino D, Pecci J, Pareja Galeano H. The effects of isokinetic training in athletes after knee surgery: A systematic review. The Physician and Sportmedicine. 2023:1-8

[12] Tsaklis P, Abatzides G. ACL rehabilitation program using a combined isokinetic and isotonic strengthening protocol. Isokinetics and Exercise Science. 2002;**10**(4):211-219

[13] Sekir U, Yildiz Y, Hazneci B, Ors F, Aydin T. Effect of isokinetic training on strength, functionality and proprioception in athletes with functional ankle instability. Knee Surgery, Sports Traumatology, Arthroscopy. 2007;**15**:654-664

[14] Zapparoli FY, Riberto M. Isokinetic evaluation of the hip flexor and extensor muscles: A systematic review. Journal of Sport Rehabilitation. 2017;**26**(6):556-566. DOI: 10.1123/jsr.2016-0036

[15] Bergamin M, Gobbo S, Bullo V, Vendramin B, Duregon F, Frizziero A, et al. Reliability of a device for the knee and ankle isometric and isokinetic strength testing in older adults. Muscles, Ligaments and Tendons Journal. 2017;7(2):323-330. DOI: 10.11138/mltj/2017.7.2.323

[16] Stark T, Walker B, Phillips JK, Fejer R, Beck R. Hand-held dynamometry correlation with the gold standard isokinetic dynamometry: A systematic review. PM & R: The Journal of Injury, Function, and Rehabilitation. 2011;**3**(5):472-479. DOI: 10.1016/j.pmrj.2010.10.025

[17] Habets B, Staal JB, Tijssen M, van Cingel R. Intrarater reliability of the Humac NORM isokinetic dynamometer for strength measurements of the knee and shoulder muscles. BMC Research Notes. 2018;**11**(1):15. DOI: 10.1186/s13104-018-3128-9

[18] Şahin Ö. Rehabilitasyonda izokinetik değerlendirmeler. Cumhuriyet Tıp Dergisi. 2010;**32**(4):386-396

[19] Muñoz-Bermejo L, Pérez-Gómez J, Manzano F, Collado-Mateo D, Villafaina S, Adsuar JC. Reliability of isokinetic knee strength measurements in children: A systematic review and meta-analysis. PLoS One. 2019;**14**(12):1-15. DOI: 10.1371/journal.pone.0226274

[20] Contreras-Díaz G, Chirosa-Ríos LJ, Chirosa-Ríos I, Intelangelo L, Jerez-Mayorga D, Martinez-Garcia D. Reliability of isokinetic hip flexor and extensor strength measurements in healthy subjects and athletes: A systematic review and meta-analysis. International Journal of Environmental Research and Public Health. 2021;**18**(21):11326-11329. DOI: 10.3390/ijerph182111326

[21] Borges O. Isometric and isokinetic knee extension and flexion torque in men and women aged 20-70. Scandinavian Journal of Rehabilitation Medicine. 1989;**21**(1):45-53

[22] Montgomery LC, Douglass LW, Deuster PA. Reliability of an isokinetic test of muscle strength and endurance. The Journal of Orthopaedic and Sports Physical Therapy. 1989;**10**(8):315-322. DOI: 10.2519/jospt.1989.10.8.315

[23] Dvir Z. Clinical applicability of isokinetics: A review. Clinical Biomechanics (Bristol, Avon). 1991;**6**(3):133-144. DOI: 10.1016/0268-0033(91)90024-K

[24] Saral I, Agirman M, Basat H, Surucu S, Mahirogullari M, Cakar E. A comparison of isokinetic muscle strength in patients with chondromalacia patella: A cross-sectional study. European Review for Medical and Pharmacological Sciences. 2022;**26**(21):7771-7778. DOI: 10.26355/eurrev_202211_30126

[25] Arhos E, Ito N, Giordana A, Nolan JRTP, Snyder-Mackler L, Silberagel KG. Who's afraid of electrical Stimülation? Let's Re-visit the application of NMES at the knee. Journal of orthopaedic sports. Physical Therapy. 2024;**54**(2):1-6

[26] Carvalho MTX, Guesser Pinheiro VH, Alberton CL. Effectiveness of neuromuscular electrical stimulation training combined with exercise on patient-reported outcomes measures in people with knee osteoarthritis: A systematic review and meta-analysis. Physiotherapy Research Internationa. 2023;**29**(1):e2062

[27] Yeşilöz Ö, Aksoy MH. The effectiveness of peroneal nerve stimulation combined with neuromuscular electrical stimulation in the management of knee osteoarthritis: A randomized controlled single-blind study. Turkish Journal of Physical Medicine and Rehabilitation. 2023;**69**(3):317

[28] Petrucci A, Guglielmino D, Pecci J, Pareja GH. The effects of isokinetic training in athletes after knee surgery: A systematic review. The Physician and Sportsmedicine, (just-accepted). 2023

[29] Akıncıoğlu B, Kocahan T. Russsian current versus high voltage current with isokinetic training on the quadriceps muscle strength and endurance. Journal of Exercise Rehabilitation. 2020;**16**(3):272

[30] AR Lucas-Toumbourou S, McCarthy B. A comparison of the analgesic efficacy of medium-frequency alternating current and TENS. Physiotherapy. 2009;**95**(4):280-288. DOI: 10.1016/j.physio Ward.2009.06.005

[31] Ward AR, Robertson AW, Sensory RVJ. Sensory, motor, and pain thresholds for stimulation with medium frequency. Alternating Current. 1998;**79**:273-278. DOI: 10.1016/S0003-9993(98)90006-5

[32] Vaz MA, Frasson VB. Low-frequency pulsed current versus kilohertz-frequency alternating currents: A scoping literatüre review. Archives of Physical Medicine and Rehabilitation. 2018;**99**(4):792-805. DOI: 10.1016/j.apmr.2017.12.001

[33] Becher M, Springer S, Braun-Benyamin O, Laufer Y. The effect of an ınterphase ınterval on electrically ınduced dorsiflexion force and fatigue in subjects with an upper motor neuron lesion. Artificial Organs. 2016;**40**(8): 778-785. DOI: 10.1111/aor.12698

[34] Baptista GB, Cardoso J, Ferreira B. Comparative analysis of the effect between FES, RUSSA, and AUSSIE therapeutic currents in individuals with hypertonia spastic post-stroke case study. British Journal of Medicine and Medical Research. 2017;**19**(8):1-9. DOI: 10.9734/BUMMER/2017/30644

[35] Lima EPF, Rodrigues GBOO. A Estımulação Russa No Fortalecımento Da Musculatura Abdomınal. ABCD. Arquivos Brasileiros de Cirurgia Digestiva (São Paulo). 2012;**25**(2):125-128 Erişim Adresi: scielo.br/j/abcd/a/XhQcdtsdPqtHr5PnQ7Bn4tc/abstract/?lang=pt

[36] Şahan N. Diz osteoartritli hastalarda quadriceps femoris kasına uygulanan iki farklı elektroterapi akımının etkilerinin karşılaştırılması. Journal of Exercise Therapy and Rehabilitation. 2020;7(2):109-118. Erişim Adresi: dergipark.org.tr/en/pub/jetr/issue/56637/577905

[37] Cittadin GL, Ansolin GZ, Furtado Santana NP, Tonini TL, Buzanello Azevedo MR, de Albuquerque CE, et al. Comparison between Russian and Aussie currents in the grip strength and thickness muscles of the non-dominant hand: A double-blind, prospective, randomized-controlled study. Turkish Journal of Physical Medicine and Rehabilitation. 2020;**66**(4):423-428. DOI: 10.5606/tftrd.2020.4718

[38] Ganesh GS, Kumari R, Pattnaik M, Mohanty P, Kaur P, Dakshinamoorthy A. Effectiveness of faradic and Russian currents on plantar flexor muscle spasticity, ankle motor recovery, and functional gait in stroke patients. Physiotherapy

Research International. 2018;**23**(2):1-8. DOI: 10.1002/pri.1705

[39] Akinoglu B, Kocahan T. Russian current versus high voltage current with isokinetic training on the quadriceps muscle strength and endurance. Journal of Exercise Rehabilitation. 2020;**16**(3):272-278. DOI: 10.12965/jer.2040260.130

[40] Dantas LO, Vieira A, Siqueira ALJ, Salvini TF, Durigan JLQ. Comparison between the effects of 4 different electrical stimulation current waveforms on isometric knee extension torque and perceived discomfort in healthy women. Muscle & Nerve. 2015;**51**(1):76-82. DOI: 10.1002/mus.24280

[41] Ward AR, Oliver WG, Buccella D. Wrist extensor torque production and discomfort associated with low-frequency and burst-modulated kilohertz-frequency currents. Physical Therapy. 2006;**86**:1360-1367

[42] Medeiros FV, Bottaro M, Vieira A, Lucas TP, Modesto KA, Bo APL, et al. Kilohertz and low-frequency electrical stimulation with the same pulse duration have similar efficiency for inducing isometric knee extension torque and discomfort. American Journal of Physical Medicine & Rehabilitation. 2017;**96**:388-394

[43] de Carvalho AR, Reginato A, Reginato GA, Schuck KSR, Neves M, Bertolini GRF. Aussie current and quadriceps muscle endurance: A randomized clinical trial. Sport Sciences for Health. 2023;**19**(2):565-572

[44] Ren Y, Yue T, Qi F. Isokinetic strength training improves motor function in a Chinese classical dancer with knee injury: A case repost. In: 2021 International Conference on Health Bih Data and Smart Sports(HBDSS). Guilin, China. 2021. pp. 60-64. DOI: 10.1109/HBDSS54392.2021.00020

[45] Nambi G. Effects of isokinetic knee muscle training on bone morphogenetic proteins and inflammatory biomarkers in post-traumatic osteoarthritis after anterior cruciate ligament injury: A randomized trial. Journal of Rehabilitation Medicine. 2020:9

[46] Lee SEK, de Lira CAB, Nouailhetas VLA, Vancini RL, Andrade MS. Do isometric, isotonic and/or isokinetic strength training produce different strength outcomes. Journal of Bodywork and Movement Therapies. 2018;**22**:430-437

[47] Ke P, Pereira KL, Stachelski RA, Azevedo MRB, De Crvallo AR, Bertolini GRF. KiloHertz currents on aspects of muscle function: A scoping review. Journal of Bodywork and Movement Therapies. 2022;**32**:110-119

Chapter 9

Health Promotion through Advanced Physical Activity Programs for Individuals with Intellectual and Developmental Disabilities

Meir Lotan and Alberto Romano

Abstract

Individuals with intellectual and developmental disabilities (IDD) present multiple co-morbidities within the medical, physiological, and mental areas, thereby putting them at an increased risk for a variety of illnesses. Moreover, many of them are living a life of inactivity, thereby worsening their health condition. Many researchers have identified a clear relationship between physical fitness and wellness. This chapter will describe the poor physical condition of individuals with IDD and will suggest some intervention possibilities, focusing on motivational factors and integration into the person's daily living routines. While some physical activity possibilities are free and can be found online, other more advanced tools for promoting an active lifestyle can be implemented with this group of people. The present chapter will suggest research-based effective strategies to enhance the physical activity of people with IDD through remote activity intervention programs, virtual reality training, and personally adapted simple training applications.

Keywords: exercise therapy, physical fitness, intellectual disability, developmental disabilities, exergaming, telerehabilitation

1. Introduction

1.1 Intellectual and developmental disability

Since 1908, intellectual and developmental disability (IDD) has been repeatedly defined by the American association of intellectual and developmental disability (AAIDD) (formerly American Association on Mental Retardation).

The definition of IDD has four main components: Developmental, mental, adaptive, and the need for care and support [1, 2]. The acceptable definition of IDD in the Western world includes the three following components:

1. Disability level in mental functioning – intelligence – refers to a general mental ability, such as learning, making conclusions, problem-solving, and others. An intellectual quotient (IQ) under 70IQ means two standard deviations below the population average and is defined as intellectual disability. Intellectual disability within the range of 55–70IQ is defined as mild IDD, within the range of 40–54IQ – moderate IDD, within the range of 25–39IQ – severe IDD, and IQ under 24IQ is defined as profound IDD [1].

2. Significant disability in adaptive behavior – adaptive behavior is a collection of conceptual, social, and practical skills learned and performed by people in everyday life. Limitation in adaptive behavior affects everyday life and the ability to cope with changes and environmental demands. In practice, this means lowering about two standard deviations from the average in standardized adaptation tests [3, 4]. These skills are distributed into three major categories:

   a. Conceptual skills: Including language and learning, time concepts, quantity concepts, self-direction, etc.

   b. Social skills: Interpersonal skills, social responsibility, self-esteem, naiveté, caution, solving social problems, ability to act according to rules, abide by laws, etc.

   c. Practical skills – activities of daily living: Self-care, occupational skills, maintaining self-health, meeting timetables/routine, safety, using money, using public transportation, using the phone, etc.

3. IDD signs first appear before age 18 [1, 5]. This definition is intended to distinguish people who are born with IDD from adults who have a cognitive disability i.e., attained at an older age against the background of various old age diseases such as Alzheimer's and the like.

Within these three categories, the four levels of intellectual disability are generally defined as follows:

- Mild IDD: People who demonstrate independence in most areas of daily living and require ad hoc support only in situations of change or crisis.

- Moderate IDD: People who need limited support in all areas of daily living, which is given regularly for short periods of time in order to learn, practice, and become competent in using all their skills.

- Severe IDD: People who need increased, regular support i.e., not limited in time in all areas of daily living in order to function actively. Without such support, individuals are unable to fulfill their basic needs.

- Profound IDD: People who need immediate support from an external support provider in fulfilling actions in all areas of daily living [6].

Therefore, IDD is a comprehensive term covering cognitive and physical limitations resulting from central nervous system dysfunction, surfacing in childhood with lifelong consequences [7].

IDD can arise from a variety of causes, encompassing genetic, environmental, and perinatal factors. Genetic mutations, either through additions, deletions, or alterations in specific genes or chromosome abnormalities, contribute significantly to the onset of IDD. Exposure to harmful substances during pregnancy, such as alcohol or infections, can adversely impact fetal development, manifesting in various cognitive and neurological impairments [8]. Moreover, preterm births, complications during childbirth, and traumatic brain injuries stand as significant contributors to the complex etiology of IDD [9].

The World Health Organization and other leading organizations within the realm of IDD perceive IDD as a dynamic phenomenon that may change over time [10]. This change derives from the understanding that a person with IDD can improve his functioning in most living areas through personally customized programs and suitable support [10]. On the other hand, an individual with IDD can demonstrate relapse in his abilities against the background of functional and medical problems, which showed higher prevalence compared to the general population [1]. Especially when severe and profound IDD is concerned, additional severe neurological and psychiatric co-morbidity is also often diagnosed, which is expressed, among others, in defects in the communicative, academic, physical, and behavioral functioning in the various environments [1, 11–14].

Co-morbidity, which characterizes this population, makes it more "fragile" than the normative population [15], with significantly increased health needs which in practice lead to relatively many hospitalizations and excessive use of drugs, the efficiency of which is not always apparent [16]. All these require the intervention of healthcare professionals [17] and providing increased customized care.

Moreover, the multiple medical needs in this population constitute a financial burden to the families and the health and welfare system [18]. Therefore, there are quite a few recommendations in the research literature to try to improve the control and therapy systems by institutionalizing multi-systemic mechanisms supported by cost-effective and efficient medical screening tools, enabling cost reduction [18].

However, as these needs are multiple, it is difficult to provide them [19]. To effectively and quickly identify whether there have been any changes in the condition of the service recipient, suitable assessment tools need to be devised. On the one hand, these tools will make it easier for direct caregivers to identify changes without increasing the load of tasks they already have, devise therapeutic programs, and advance all adaptive areas, and on the other hand, they will allow wise allocation of existing health resources [20]. At the same time, the approach that direct caregivers should be consulted when making therapeutic changes is increasingly rooted [21].

1.2 Unmet therapeutic needs

Equity in healthcare should be a minimum standard for everyone in all countries. However, despite existing evidence in the literature regarding the ill health of individuals with IDD, this minority group still suffers disproportionately and to an unnecessary degree [22]. Given their more complex needs, one might anticipate that individuals with IDD would receive increased assistance from mainstream services. Paradoxically, however, accessing these services can prove challenging for them, and mainstream providers may struggle to customize their care to suit their unique needs. Unfortunately, this situation has occasionally resulted in healthcare disparities for people with IDD [23]. Moreover, many authors suggest a lack of adequate health screening and preventative care in this population. Co-morbidities among adults with IDD are high and increase with age; environmental risks, however, much like those found in the population at large, such as lack of physical activity (PA) combined with inappropriate nutrition resulting in overweight and obesity, are prevalent. However, these risk factors are modifiable and preventable, and if addressed appropriately, they could lead to an enhanced overall health status within the population of individuals with IDD [24]. In order to prevent complications associated with the disabilities associated with IDD, there is a need for a comprehensive and preventive therapeutic intervention. Such therapeutic approaches should include physical therapy and hydrotherapy (to improve mobility and cardio-vascular fitness, reduce spasticity, and prevent physical deformations), occupational therapy (to enhance function within activities of daily living and attend to sensory dysfunctions), speech therapy (to enhance communication skills and improve eating abilities), special education teachers (gain computer access, enhance education, literacy skills, and social skills), music therapy (for self-expression and emotional well-being), and more. Therefore, it is in the hands of healthcare from all professions to enhance care for our clients with IDD, establishing better and intensified evaluation and therapeutic interventions to answer their needs.

1.3 Physical activity of people with IDD

Numerous investigations have indicated that consistent engagement in PA, sports, and exercise contributes to enhanced physical (i.e., balance and muscle strength) and psychosocial health and quality of life among individuals with IDD [25–29] but failed to impact the body mass index and body composition parameters. The main effects of PA for individuals with IDD were repeatedly confirmed in the literature through meta-analysis, as summarized in **Table 1**.

However, despite the essential nature of PA for this population, it was overlooked in national PA guidelines and public health recommendations until 2020, when the revised PA guidelines from the World Health Organization (WHO) explicitly included mention of people with an IDD, marking the first acknowledgment of this population in such guidelines [25].

Nevertheless, while at least 150 minutes of exercise per week for adults aged 18 to 64 [26], individuals with IDD are believed to participate in comparatively fewer PA, posing challenges in achieving optimal health [27]. Research indicates that individuals with IDD participate in only 17.5–33% of the recommended PA levels [27]. Consequently, this population has a higher obesity rate and lower physical fitness and cardiovascular endurance [28] compared to their counterparts without IDD. In addition, adults with IDD exhibit a declining PA rate, leading to sedentary behavior and an increased risk of fatigue-related diseases, low fitness levels, and obesity [29, 38]. This emphasizes the importance of addressing physical inactivity early in life to mitigate the risk of long-term health issues [39]. Moreover, sedentary lifestyles and a lack of engagement in PA contribute significantly to the substantial lifetime costs associated with health and non-healthcare services related to IDD [40]. This economic burden, coupled with the need for lifelong treatment and services, highlights the importance of addressing PA levels in individuals with IDD.

Despite the well-established health benefits of PA, reports indicate that elevating this population's PA levels may be challenging and require time to become effective [41]. Numerous personal, family, social, financial, and environmental obstacles impede the engagement of individuals with IDD in PA [42].

Personal barriers to PA for people with IDD include specific and generic health problems associated with IDD (e.g., being overweight, heart issues, unpleasant body

DOI: http://dx.doi.org/10.5772/intechopen.1004856

Reference	Aim	No. of included papers and subjects (age range)	Included levels of IDD	Included trainings	Main findings related to people with IDD
Kapsal et al. [30]	To synthesize the literature and quantify the effects of PA on the physical and psychosocial health of youth with intellectual disabilities.	109 papers, 4200 subjects (age range: 5–19.9y).	32.3% mild; 30.3% mild and moderate; 11.6% moderate; 0.6% severe/profound; 25.2% not reported.	Aerobic training, resistance training, movement/sport skills training, general physical education/activity, and balance/core stability.	PA had a large positive effect on reaction time (ES = 1.13, 95% CI 0.69–1.58), flexibility (ES = 0.91, 95% CI 0.74–1.08), and movement/sport skills (ES = 0.81, 95% CI 0.67–0.96). A moderate effect was observed for cardiovascular/cardiorespiratory fitness (ES = 0.79, 95% CI 0.69–0.94), muscular strength/endurance (ES = 0.78, 95% CI 0.64–0.91), physical functioning (ES = 0.66, 95% CI 0.43–0.90), balance/core stability (ES = 0.68, 95% CI 0.45–0.91), and physiological outcomes (ES = 0.51, 95% CI 0.42–0.69). No effect of PA was observed for BMI (ES = 0.035, p = 0.403). PA had a large effect on psychological (ES = 0.754, 95% CI 0.461–1.048), behavioral (ES = 0.986, 95% CI 0.654–1.319), and social (0.723, 95% CI 0.443–1.002) outcomes. A moderate effect was reported for cognitive outcomes (ES = 0.534, 95% CI 0.239–0.829). No effect was found for emotional outcomes (ES = 0.249, 95% CI -0.201-0.699).
Jeng et al. [31]	To determine whether exercise training improves skill-related fitness in adolescents with IDD.	14 papers, 386 subjects (age range: 13.6–18.8y).	57.1% mild; 21.4% mild and moderate; 14.4% moderate; 7.1% moderate and severe/profound.	Circuit training, muscle strengthening, unified sports, hippo therapy, Swiss ball exercise, traditional Greek dancing treadmill and Wii Sports game training, sensorimotor training, device-assisted training, water aerobic exercise, low-intensity run/walk training, aerobic dance, walking exercise, Taekwondo, adapted dancing, road-running training, and horseback-riding machine training.	Exercise training has positive moderate to large effects on agility (ES = 0.781, 95% CI 1.279–0.284), power (ES = 0.760, 95% CI 0.441–1.080), reaction time to light (ES = 1.465, 95% CI 2.433–0.497), and sound cues (ES = 1.286, 95% CI 1.735–0.838), and speed (ES = 0.526, 95% CI 0.835–0.218). No effect was found for static (ES = 0.82, 95% CI -2.12 – 0.48) and dynamic balance on the balance beam (ES = −0.73, 95% CI -1.55 – 0.09).

Reference	Aim	No. of included papers and subjects (age range)	Included levels of IDD	Included trainings	Main findings related to people with IDD
Shin & Park [32]	To synthesize the effects of physical exercise programs on individuals with ID	14 papers, N/R subjects (means range: 8.5–60.9y).	N/R The authors reported that they included *"participants with IDD, except for diagnoses of Down syndrome, Prader-Willi syndrome, Rett syndrome, and Williams syndrome."*	Rhythmic gymnastics programs, balance and muscle strength exercises, exercise/training programs, aerobic exercise programs, physical fitness programs, endurance training, health promotion programs, self-directed strength training, PA interventions, and school-based cardiovascular fitness.	Exercise programs had large positive effects on self-esteem (ES = 0.910, 95% CI 0.75–1.08), force (ES = 1.190, 95% CI 0.62–1.78), balance (ES = 1.150, 95% CI 0.68–1.61), pulmonary ventilation (ES = 0.816, 95% CI 0.03–1.61), and other physiological measures (not specified) (ES = 2.180, 95% CI 1.17–3.18). A moderate effect was observed for BMI (ES = −0.649, 95% CI -0.83 – −0.47) and VO2 peak (ES = 0.422, 95% CI 0.21–0.63). No effect was observed for the weight (ES = −0.02, 95% CI -0.34 – 0.29), body fat (ES = 0.12, 95% CI -0.15 – 0.40), lean mass (ES = 0.023, 95% CI -0.30 – 0.76), and heart rate (ES = 0.08, 95% CI -0.23 – 0.39).
St. John, Borschneck, & Cairney [33]	To assess the effectiveness of exercise interventions based on experimental designs on individuals with IDD.	18 papers, 799 subjects (age range: N/R).	34.9% mild and moderate; 4.6% severe/ profound; 16.3% Down syndrome; 44.2% not reported.	N/R The authors reported, "The intervention must have been one that was specific to exercise. Any and all programs were included regardless of setting."	Exercise programs had large effects on balance (ES = 1.25, 95% CI 0.39–2.90) and lower body musculoskeletal strength (ES = 0.86, 95% CI 0.30–1.42). A moderate effect was observed for the upper body musculoskeletal strength (ES = 0.55, 95% CI 0.17–1.26). No effect was observed for aerobic fitness (ES = 0.13, 95% CI -0.11 – 0.37), flexibility (ES = −0.19, 95% CI -1.73 – 1.34), and step count (ES = 0.30, 95% CI -0.15 – 0.75).
Maïano et al. [34]	To examine the effects of exercise interventions designed to improve balance in young people with intellectual disabilities.	15 papers, 403 subjects (age range: 8–25y).	60.0% mild; 26.7% mild and moderate; 6.7% moderate; 6.6% not reported.	Balance exercises, strength exercises, computerized balance exercises, creative dance activities, hippotherapy exercises, rope-skipping exercises, Swiss ball exercises, tai chi exercises, and trampolines.	Exercise programs had a large effect on static balance (ES = 0.82, 95% CI 0.46–1.18). A moderate effect was found for dynamic balance (ES = 0.79, 95% CI 0.11–1.46).

Reference	Aim	No. of included papers and subjects (age range)	Included levels of IDD	Included trainings	Main findings related to people with IDD
Obrusnikova, Firkin, & Farquhar [35]	To review clinical trials that evaluated the effects of aerobic exercise interventions on cardiorespiratory fitness in adults with IDD.	16 papers, 549 subjects (age range: 21–58y).	43.8% mild and moderate; 6.2% moderate and severe/ profound; 6.2% mild to severe/profound 43.8% not reported.	Aerobic exercise and aerobic exercise combined with resistance, balance, or flexibility training.	Aerobic exercise interventions had a moderate effect on cardiorespiratory fitness (ES = 0.44, 95% CI 0.22–0.66), 6MWT (ES = 0.48, 95% CI 0.14–0.83, and both absolute (ES = 0.57, 95% CI 0.30–0.84) and relative (ES = 0.50, 95% CI 0.20–0.80) VO2 peak.
Harris et al. [36]	To review the randomized controlled trials on the effects of PA interventions to prevent weight gain in young adults with IDD.	6 papers, 178 subjects (age range: 10–30y).	83.3% mild and moderate; 16.7% not reported.	Bicycle ergometer and aerobic training, strength and endurance training, conditioning and plyometric jumps training, whole-body vibration and isometric exercise, aerobic treadmill ergometer, and aerobic rowing ergometer intervention.	No effect of PA was observed for body weight (ES = 0.45, 95% CI -1.04 – 0.72), BMI (ES = 0.29, 95% CI -0.64 – 0.51), waist circumference (ES = 1.47, 95% CI -4.03 – 1.75), percentage body fat (ES = 0.81, 95% CI -2.03 – 1.15), fat mass (ES = 0.68, 95% CI -1.60 – 1.08), and lean mass (ES = 0.43, 95% CI -0.08 – 1.62).
Yang, Liang, & Hui-Ping Sit [37]	To determine the effects of PA on mental health, including psychological health and cognitive function, in children and adolescents with IDD.	15 papers, 630 subjects (age range: 5-17y)	26.7% mild; 5.3% mild and moderate; 20% not reported.	Competitive sports, non-competitive sports, cognitive exercise, therapeutic exercise, and aerobic exercise.	PA has a large effect on overall mental health (ES = 0.90, 95% CI 0.66–1.14) and cognitive function (ES = 1.24, 95% CI 0.87–1.60). A moderate effect was found for psychological health (ES = 0.54, 95% CI 0.37–0.71).

Abbreviation list: IDD = Intellectual and developmental disability; y = Years; PA = Physical activity; ES = Effect size; CI = Confidence interval; BMI = Body mass index; N/R = Not reported; VO_2 *= Oxygen volume; 6MWT = Six-minute walking test.*

Table 1.
Synthesis of recent meta-analyses investigating the effect of PA and exercise training on physical, physiological, and psychological outcomes in children and adults with IDD.

feelings, etc.), the lack of motivation toward PA, the physical and intellectual disabilities of the participants, and the presence of behavioral problems. Interestingly, PA itself may positively influence many of such personal barriers. For instance, consistent engagement in regular physical exercise enhances aerobic endurance, cardiovascular capacity, flexibility, and agility while reducing adipose mass in people with IDD [43]. Furthermore, joining PA has been reported as a strategy to mitigate and diminish negative behaviors [44] and to increase the motor functional level of people with IDD [45]. The mutual influence of PA on its barriers and vice-versa may generate virtuous (if performing PA simplifies the barriers overcome) or vicious (if the barriers limit the engagement in PA) circles. Individuating and using personal motivational factors to enhance the willingness of people with IDD to participate in PA may help in promoting a virtuous circle to establish. Performing PA in a group or within social interactive situations (e.g., involvement of peers with and without IDD, socialization moments, etc.), together with the provision of positive reinforcement for participation (e.g., being rewarded and praised, receiving medals and prizes, etc.), have been reported as facilitators for participation in PA [46, 47]. Moreover, personal factors such as the desire to look and feel good, determination to succeed, and a good understanding and knowledge of the benefits associated with PA act as facilitators for the involvement of individuals with IDD [46, 47]. This highlights the need for an explanation of the benefits of PA to people with IDD who often lack knowledge about maintaining a healthy lifestyle. These elements must be taken into high consideration when planning to enhance the PA level of an individual with IDD.

Furthermore, it was reported that an increased level of intellectual disability severity, along with the associated requirement for supervision, represents a constraint on engaging in PA [48]. Accordingly, Sundblom and coauthors [48] assert that the level of intellectual disability determines the PA intervention feasibility and the method of delivering it. In fact, due to the wide range of functional levels and complex needs shown by people with IDD and their families, highly individualized intervention programs are required to achieve behavioral change and promote PA in the population with IDD. Preliminary evidence in the field pointed out the importance of adapting the PA program to the individuals' needs, incorporating it into their daily routine, and involving the individuals' caregivers and environments [49–52]. Daily routine integration may require a prolonged period of time before becoming effective, as people with IDD tend to resist modifications to their habits [44]. However, when an effective integration of the PA program into the daily routine is established, it could play as a facilitator in engagement in PA. Furthermore, Kapsal et al. [30], in their meta-analysis, remarked on the critical importance of the social nature of PA, suggesting that engaging in PA in groups may prove more beneficial for individuals with IDD (a table presenting the effectiveness of PA programs for individuals with IDD is presented as an appendix at the end of the current chapter (appendix 1).

Besides personal factors, several environmental factors may act as facilitators and barriers to PA and healthcare in general for people with IDD.

1.4 Obstacles to better care by the health system for a person with IDD

According to the literature, the factors limiting the quality of care for people with IDD within the health systems are several and were briefly presented below:

- Challenging communication – The difficulty in understanding the subjective condition of a person with IDD and gathering information regarding his medical background makes it difficult for health professionals to determine a correct anamnesis and needs. Unclear anamnesis is one of the factors preventing people with IDD from getting the best healthcare they need. Some individuals with IDD are unable to speak at all, which makes it difficult to identify symptoms and illnesses; these people will also have difficulty expressing pain and asking for help [53].

- Lack of cooperation on the part of individuals with IDD – Some with IDD are uncomfortable in unfamiliar situations and with unfamiliar people. Sometimes, it is impossible to explain to the person with IDD the importance of PA or medical procedures that may be painful/unpleasant, such as physical efforts, taking blood, measuring weight, and using various medical tools.

- Unconventional etiology and complex medical symptoms – In some cases, the etiology of diseases in individuals with IDD differs from that in neurotypical individuals. Such differences, or a combination of several diseases that present different symptoms simultaneously, make it difficult for the healthcare professional to locate the source of the disease. Moreover, individuals with IDD sometimes present a complex of several diseases and symptoms in one patient that can complicate and delay the treatment for that person [54].

- Lack of professional knowledge of the healthcare staff – The complexity and specific nature of medical conditions and symptoms require additional knowledge by the healthcare staff on top of the knowledge needed when treating a client within the general population. Despite this, in general, the knowledge and training of health professionals on issues related to IDD are lacking around the world. Therefore, it is unrealistic to expect a healthcare professional to be familiar with specific symptoms and signs associated with IDD [55].

- Service providers' attitudes toward people with developmental disabilities – Some argue that this reason is the most challenging barrier [56]. A study that surveyed nurses' attitudes about providing care to individuals with IDD found that more than 30% of respondents reported feeling uncomfortable carrying out health-promoting activities with individuals with IDD. When asked if they enjoy treating these patients like others, 22.9% said no. When asked whether they would like to transfer these patients to another caregiver, 12.5% answered yes [56].

- Tenure and experience of the treatment staff of individuals with IDD – In large health clinics, employee turnover is frequent. The tenure of the treating staff is essential for those with special needs. Staff permanence is important in light of medical problems and conditions that require good familiarity with the person with IDD and the establishment of therapist-patient relationships with proper rapport that enable ongoing and continuous treatment to be performed. With specific reference to PA, limited staff, the lack of instructors expert at adapted PA, and low level of interest of the staff in PA were reported as barriers to PA in people with IDD [46].

- Opinions of the individuals with IDD – Individuals with IDD were interviewed and asked about their preferences. They indicated that they preferred a doctor who is experienced in treating individuals with IDD over a more professional doctor [57]. This aspect emphasizes the need for experienced staff able to create an effective and empathetic therapeutic relationship with the person with IDD.

- Ethical issues and lack of specific procedures for individuals with IDD – When treating individuals with IDD, very complicated ethical problems arise regarding medical decision-making and agreement on the treatment plan by the therapists or by the person himself [58]. There are medical procedures that require the patient's cooperation, which may be challenging to obtain from an individual with IDD. In such cases, special procedures can prevent unnecessary suffering of the client. In addition, since the staff treating an individual with IDD is more complex than is usually the norm, especially among residents living in the residential facilities, more factors, and related individuals (staff and family members) are involved in the decision-making process in a way that goes beyond the usual process for an individual without IDD.

- Accessibility problems and environmental limitations – The environment in health facilities is not always suitable and accessible for individuals with IDD, limiting their access to PA and facilities. Issues like the presence of architectural barriers, the absence of adapted facilities (such as gyms and sports centers), and community support (e.g., transportation services), burden the people with IDD and their caregivers [46]. Physical accessibility requires elevators, ramps, cranes, and wide passages. In addition, the accessibility of the treatment also includes special adjustments such as a variety of means of communication according to the types of disabilities [56].

- Financing – Individuals with special needs usually suffer from many problems, including heavy economic costs. Various health treatments and accessing PA services are not their top priority, especially when these treatments are not funded or subsidized by the state. In addition, treatment for this population requires a longer time than regular treatments due to the need to perform specific demonstrations and explanations.

- Unlike people in the general population, individuals with IDD do not always know their options and rights. As a result, they depend on family, housing, and healthcare staff who care for them. Organizing the PA program in a way that allows everyone around the person with IDD to participate without too many sacrifices in terms of time may enable a higher participation rate in PA. This concept emphasizes the need for the involvement of caregivers in planning the healthcare path in general and the PA program specifically.

In accordance with the difficulties arising from the literature on the medical treatment of this population, it was found at the same time that the current health condition of people with IDD is deficient.

In the 30s of the previous millennium, the mean age at death for people with IDD was about 19 years; in the 1970s, this number rose to about 59 years; in the 1990s, to 66 years; and today, it is close to general life expectancy. For instance, the mean age at death for Down syndrome (DS) was 9 years in the 1920s and 56 years today [59]. Advancements in medical technology and heightened social awareness during the twentieth century have contributed to this remarkable increase in lifespan. Historically, many individuals with IDD faced premature mortality due to associated medical complications, congenital anomalies, and infections. This semi-positive trend should be further improved by updating assessment and therapeutic efforts until individuals with IDD receive up-to-date medical and habilitative support adapted to current medical facilities and their multiple medical and functional needs.

The present chapter explores new and up-to-date assessments and therapeutic possibilities for individuals with IDD with the intent of such technologies to become common practice in the treatment of individuals with IDD.

2. Evaluation

Since IDD is defined as a dynamic situation, adults with IDD it is to have the functioning level of this group of clients assessed once a period (depending on the guidelines by the authorities). However, the shortage in therapeutic services and other barriers mentioned earlier within the current chapter make such evaluation an unmet burden for the managing healthcare professionals. Moreover, the complexity of medical conditions presented by individuals with IDD and the complexity of existing assessment tools makes it impossible to meet such demands without increasing the load of tasks the healthcare providers already have [12, 57]. Therefore, meeting these demands necessitates constructing new and comprehensive assessment tools available online and easy enough to be used by direct care providers [21]. Such an approach will make it easier for direct caregivers to identify changes without increasing the load of tasks they already have, devise therapeutic programs, and advance all adaptive areas. On the other hand, they will allow wise allocation of existing health resources [20].

Due to the difficulties mentioned, we constructed a new scale, the Functional Screening Tool for Adults with Intellectual and Developmental Disabilities (FST-IDD). The new screening tool has been built as an online tool based on existing questionnaires and following the most up-to-date IDD definitions by AAIDD and the WHO. The tool was examined and found to be valid, reliable, and sensitive. It also has high psychometric values for quick detection of changes in the functioning of adult service recipients with IDD. This new scale was published in a series of articles [60–62] and can be found and used to enhance periodical evaluations of individuals with IDD who are under the reader's care.

3. Therapeutic intervention

3.1 Embedding exercise routines in daily situations

The caregivers of the individual with IDD should not be limited to relying on health-related disciplines, and the therapeutic intervention should not be limited to what is administered in the treatment room or during individually applied sessions (direct therapy/hands-on). In order to attain a continuous effect, therapists and caregivers should cooperate with the care providers and families to construct a comprehensive intervention that taps into natural resources and intertwines within daily activities and situations. Many have asserted that an activation program taught to caregivers/families was highly recommended throughout the life of the individual with IDD, and regular activity was recommended for this population's long-lasting health status [63].

It is therefore recommended that caregivers implement an exercise plan in order to construct a supportive network around the client. Such day-by-day and hour-by-hour support will allow everyone involved in caring for the individual with IDD to be aware of his\her needs and, therefore, construct and support a supplementary management program. One such program reported in the past by the first author is a physical intervention program that meets many positive aspects. It has been running in a residential center for about 20 years with a group of young individuals with DS now aged 32–35 years. Since adolescence, this group has participated in movement and music recreation activities. Using the artistic product of this activity, they started to present a show that presented their drumming and dancing skills within their residential center on holidays and special occasions. As time went by, their achievements led to a growing interest in their performance by external organizations, leading to a steady stream of requests for external performances. In order to respond to the growing demand and upgrade their professional performance, the group now meets for three 2-hour practice sessions a week, with increasing practice intensity before performance dates. Over the past 4 years, a cohort of healthy children from a conventional school has been seamlessly integrated into the existing group of DS dancers [19].

The program's benefit lies in incorporating intense, high-level PA several times per week, intertwined with the outgoing/happy nature of individuals with DS; it holds a strong motivation appeal (no dropouts over 20 years). The program's success suggests that when a program's motivational aspects are high enough, even individuals with DS who usually prefer a sedentary lifestyle can maintain a continuous healthy and active life.

The concept and outcome of this program correspond with the authors who claim that creative aspects, such as music, movement, and dance, can significantly affect the development of individuals with IDD and their adherence to exercise programs such as the one described above [64]. In this example, the later inclusion of a group of healthy dancers/singers enabled the participants with IDD to further expose their friendly, outgoing nature. It spiced up their performance while corresponding with recommendations of the WHO [65] and the United Nations [66] regarding the need for community participation of individuals with IDD within the general population.

3.2 A few words on motivation

Motivated individuals will be engaged with activities, persist with challenging tasks, believe themselves competent, see success as within their control, and experience pleasure when they succeed. Early motivation predicts later success in typically developing children [67] and children with IDD [68].

Nevertheless, individuals with IDD have been shown to present motivational deficits [69, 70]. Some studies suggest that when performing physical and recreational activities, individuals with IDD were found to be less involved in actually engaging in activities than their typically developing peers less involved [71].

The finding of a vast literature review regarding the motivation of individuals with IDD supports the notion that social factors (e.g., peer modeling) together with environmental factors (e.g., audio and audio-visual reinforcements) may be effective in initiating and maintaining participation of individuals with IDD in prolonged PA programs essential for their health and well-being [72]. One way to increase motivation to participate in and adhere to PA programs is by using exciting and appealing techniques. Therefore, the next part of the chapter will present a few settings and techniques that were found effective in enhancing the participation of individuals with IDD in PA programs.

4. Exciting new technologies

4.1 Telerehabilitation

Telerehabilitation refers to providing rehabilitation services through telecommunication technology, such as video conferencing, mobile applications, and other digital platforms [73]. This approach has gained significant attention and adoption, especially in light of the COVID-19 pandemic, which has limited in-person services in many settings. The WHO and the World Bank [74], in their co-produced World Report on Disability, concluded that there is growing evidence supporting the efficacy and effectiveness of telerehabilitation and confirmed the efficacy of remote rehabilitation as an effective service delivery model for rehabilitation professionals (i.e., telerehabilitation).

Preliminary reports suggest the positive effect of such intervention mode for delivering health services for children and adults with IDD [75–78], autism spectrum disorder [79, 80], and for addressing communicational needs of young children with severe neurodevelopmental disabilities [81, 82]. Moreover, several comparative studies concluded that there is no significant difference in clinical outcomes between in-person health services and those achieved through telerehabilitation [83–86].

Telerehabilitation offers several potential benefits for the care of people with IDD and their families, including:

- Accessibility – Telerehabilitation can increase access to services for individuals with IDD, especially those in remote or underserved areas where specialized services might not be readily available, preventing unnecessary delays in care and support, and facilitating early intervention [87, 88].

- Continuity of care – Telerehabilitation can facilitate ongoing monitoring and support, ensuring that individuals with IDD receive consistent care and intervention over time [89].

- Convenience – Telehealth eliminates the need for travel for individuals with IDD and their families, which can be particularly challenging for those with mobility issues or transportation barriers [90].

- Customization – Telerehabilitation interventions can be tailored to meet the unique needs of individuals with IDD and their families. A combination of multiple telerehabilitation strategies (e.g., integration of video calls, videos and photos exchange and discussion, web-based monitoring tools, parent coaching with and without the person with IDD, direct activity with the person, and others) may be needed to provide the required support.

- A window into the patient's daily living environment – As telerehabilitation sessions can occur virtually everywhere and participants involved in such interventions often connect from their houses, telerehabilitation offers the professional a unique occasion to observe and assess the person's daily living environment, facilitating the provision of activity programs better intertwined into the person's daily routine.

- Collaboration – Telerehabilitation simplifies communication and information exchange between the people involved in the patient's care, facilitating meetings between the person with IDD, parents, and clinicians, as well as between clinicians themselves [89].

Telerehabilitation aimed at improving the PA of people with IDD involves using digital platforms and technologies to remotely deliver personalized exercise programs, therapeutic interventions, and PA support. This approach seeks to enhance the physical health, motor skills, functional abilities, and overall well-being of individuals with IDD, leveraging the convenience and accessibility of telehealth solutions. Here (and depicted in **Figure 1**) are some specific aspects to consider when planning a telerehabilitation program aimed at enhancing the PA of people with IDD:

- Ecological exercise programs – Remotely provided exercise programs should be constructed based on the family's daily routines and habits, aiming to integrate the program's activities into the person's living environment. PA integration into daily living tasks supports their performance [91] and helps to build the activity's significance and a new and more active routine.

- Individualized program – The activity program should be highly individualized at several levels. Activity sessions duration and intensity, type of activity, and level of provided support should be planned based on the person's attitude and physical and cognitive characteristics. The program goals setting should involve the family and, where possible, the person with IDD. The set goals must be realistic and attainable. Remote meeting planning should be regulated by mediating between the family's availability and needs for support and supervision. Moreover, the health professional should choose the most indicated support strategy for the specific case. Each of these aspects should be monitored and eventually modified during the program implementation if needed [45].

- Progress monitoring and evaluation – Establishing mechanisms for monitoring progress, tracking outcomes, and evaluating the effectiveness of telerehabilitation interventions is essential to identify areas for improvement, make data-driven decisions, provide timely and meaningful feedback, and optimize the delivery of PA support and services for individuals with IDD.

- Motivation – The motivation level of the people with IDD and their families should be taken under strict monitoring in order to maintain a high level of adherence to the program. Motivational support may be provided by preventively individuating (together with the family members) the person's motivational factors and integrating them into the activity program to enhance engagement and adherence to PA routines [77]. Moreover, progress tracking with emphasis on reached improvement (even if small) and a positive attitude of the health professional could support the family members' motivation. Furthermore, the health professional's availability to listen and welcome the reported difficulties by discussing the possible solutions with the family members could support their feelings toward the proposed program [76].

- Family and caregiver involvement – As already highlighted, involving family members, caregivers, and support staff in the telerehabilitation process can

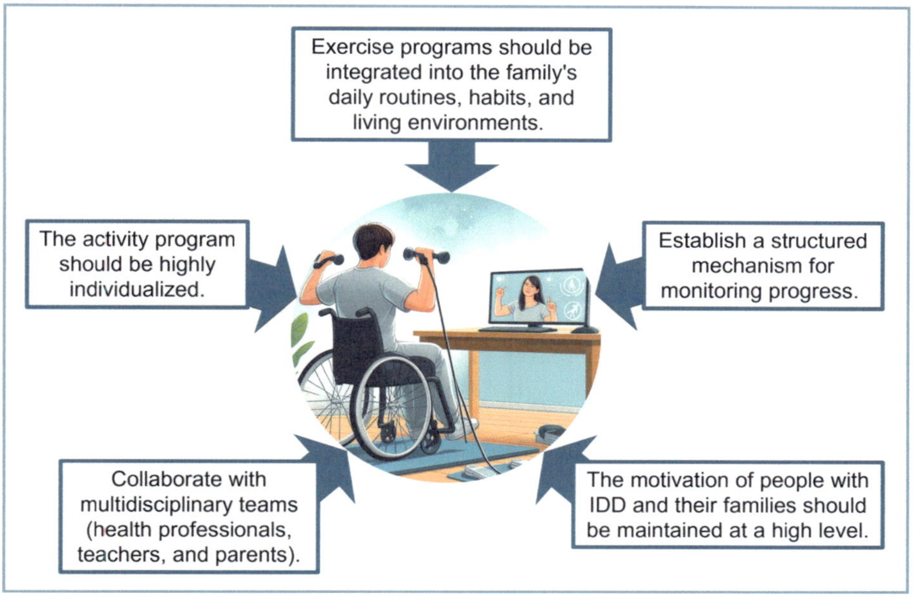

Figure 1.
Key points to consider when planning a telerehabilitation program to enhance the PA of people with IDD.

help to facilitate participation, provide additional support and supervision, and promote consistency in implementing PA programs and strategies in various settings, including home, community, and recreational environments [92].

- Multidisciplinary collaboration – Collaborating with multidisciplinary teams, including physiotherapists, occupational therapists, special educators, and other healthcare professionals, can help to ensure comprehensive assessment, planning, and delivery of PA interventions tailored to the unique needs and goals of individuals with IDD receiving telerehabilitation services.

In summary, telerehabilitation holds promise as a valuable and accessible modality for delivering health services to people with IDD, including those aimed at enhancing their PA level, reducing sedentary behaviors, leveraging technology to deliver personalized, accessible, and inclusive interventions tailored to the unique needs and preferences of this population. However, careful planning, individualization, collaboration, and ongoing evaluation are essential to address this population's unique needs and challenges and ensure the provision of high-quality, person- and family-centered care through telehealth platforms. Moreover, telerehabilitation allows for increasing the frequency and intensity of activity programs, providing individualized activities in a comfortable and familiar environment for the person. It also enables monitoring and evaluating the person's needs and progress, stimulating motivation, achieving better satisfaction, and potentially reducing service costs.

4.2 Virtual reality

Since the mid-1990s, daily life for many adults within the general population has become permeated with technology-driven activities, primarily due to the wide availability of mobile devices and low-cost personal computers that can run relevant software for various rehabilitation populations and purposes (e.g., [93]). Virtual game technology, and, more specifically, virtual reality (VR) gaming, has become commonplace, and it is now part of a clinician's repertoire of available rehabilitative tools. As numerous clinicians and researchers continue to examine ways to increase PA participation and reduce the sedentary lifestyle of individuals with IDD [94], virtual game technology represents a new means of achieving such goals.

VR gaming may be described as using computer-based interactive simulations to present users with practice opportunities for engaging in realistic activities through artificial environments [95, 96]. Virtual games provide players with an experience in two- or three-dimensional simulated virtual environments (VEs) with which they can interact and respond at different levels of motor and cognitive ability to perform tasks that are motivating, meaningful, and purposeful [97–101].

In their review of various virtual reality rehabilitation applications for people with IDD, [102] supportively concluded that those few empirical studies that have examined VE use for people with IDD have shown it to be potentially effective and meaningful. Therefore, VR may have a role in removing the barriers that impede participation and rehabilitation for people with IDD.

Our experience suggests that VR. Gaming helps to enhance physical fitness in individuals with IDD [12, 103], and it is a means to enhance participation in leisure activities [104] and improve balance with the intent of reducing falls among individuals with IDD [105].

Moreover, to date, several VEs have been used for people with IDD, permitting an examination of the potential of VR and virtual games for teaching life skills, such as route learning [106], street crossing [107], preparation for giving witness evidence in a court of law [108], coping during natural disasters such as earthquakes [109], shopping [100], improving physical fitness [12, 103], augmenting sensorimotor functioning [110], and increasing cognitive skills, such as assessing sequential time passage [111] and spatial perception [112]. Other researchers have studied the practicality of VEs for social skills training [98, 113] and as a medium for leisure activities [104, 114].

Findings from research projects across the globe [12, 103, 115] suggest that virtual gaming addresses concerns regarding the poor physical and medical challenges of individuals with IDD. As was found by many, the ability of virtual gaming to motivate individuals with IDD and to promote their cooperation, involvement, and enjoyment of PA is likely to play an essential role in helping these individuals become more physically active [12, 103, 116, 117]. Therefore, the use of VR with individuals with IDD is highly recommended.

4.3 Therapeutic snoezelen intervention, a multi-sensory approach

We live our lives through our senses. It is by means of experiencing the senses that we develop an understanding of our body and, through it, about our environment [118]. Any medical problem that a person may exhibit, which will disturb his interaction with the environment, may influence his understanding and, as a result, may disturb his development, interactions, and participation. According to Longhorn [119], without sensation and awakening of the senses, people confronted with intellectual and functional challenges will find it very difficult to understand the world around them. As a result, they will have difficulty participating, learning, and functioning. The multi-sensory approach tries to find significance in the world through an adapted sensory environment and the help of an enabling therapist. This environment awakens the client's interest, encouraging exploration and discovery of his surroundings. This exploration acts as a stepping-stone toward learning and development.

Mostly, people with IDD cannot create their own optimal environment, so it is up to us to do so. By providing a multi-sensory environment (MSE), we create a sheltered sensory experience for the client to explore. In this chapter section, we will review the benefits of an MSE called Snoezelen. The Snoezelen idea was initially designed in the 1970s in Holland and was mainly designed for people diagnosed with IDD. Snoezelen is a controlled MSE transmitting sensory stimulation through light effects, colors, sounds, music, scents, and all the combinations of different materials that can be explored with the senses and without verbal communication. So, therefore, Snoezelen can be a very helpful non-directive therapy for people with profound IDD [120]. The word Snoezelen combines two Dutch words: To doze and to sniff like a dog. The word doze indicates that a restful activity is involved, and the sniffing gives it a more sensory and dynamic aspect. The multi-sensory room is partially lit and provides sensory stimulation to the client and the therapist. The senses (such as hearing and sight, touch, taste, and smell) are provided harmoniously, whether alone or combined. They are provided according to the client's choice. The treatment aims to find a balance between relaxation and activity within the framework of a safe, adapted environment by means of an enabling therapist [121].

When considering a suitable intervention program for the client with IDD, we reviewed the suggestions of experts in the field of IDD:

- close interpersonal contact [122];
- a quiet and reassuring environment may achieve a reduction in anxiety and agitation in individuals with IDD [123];
- music is of utmost value [124, 125];
- the child will respond best to gentle, loving care, which encourages activity in an interesting but quiet environment [126];
- encourage and facilitate learning without pressuring the person;
- provide face-to-face contact, talking, singing, and touching;
- comfort the person and allow withdrawal during agitation;
- encourage active supervised movement in soft play;
- provide gentle movement of limbs and joints through their full range [127].

All the above suggestions are an integral part of the MSE, making it a preferred intervention method for children, adolescents, and adults with IDD.

Despite its widespread use, relatively few research studies have examined this method's efficiency. This is mainly the result of the fear expressed by the original founders that such exposure would eliminate the relaxed and intuitive nature of the experiential ambiance, which is crucial to the Snoezelen concept. In addition, most of the existing studies to date are based on anecdotal reports.

Therefore, the authors of the current chapter constructed a structured approach enabling systematic data gathering without harming the original cornerstones of the original concept of the Snoezelen.

Using the therapeutic snoezelen intervention (TSI) approach, the interaction within the Snoezelen environment is performed with accordance to the original concept of the Snoezelen: E.g., an adapted surrounding (set according to each client's preferences and changed following new requests or signals by the client), an enabling facilitator (constantly observing the client, monitoring their signals and mediating their intervention accordingly), and an interaction were "nothing is demanded from the clients and everything is allowed" [128]. At the same time, pre-determined information regarding the client's behaviors/challenges (i.e., How many times he took off his clothes, how many times he fell, and how many times he hit himself or others) is collected and compared with the same measures during the pre-Snoezelen intervention by the care-providers.

According to our analysis, elements contributing to the success of the TSI included [129]:

1. choosing high-quality personnel as therapists;

2. specifying target population by consulting with team members;

3. reducing the anxiety at first encounters;

4. provide a careful and organized training program for each Snoezelen/therapist;

5. pre-setting measurable therapeutic goals for each client;

6. systematic data gathering by the care providers' staff;

7. systematic implementation of intervention several times per week;

8. systematic follow-up evaluations within the natural surroundings by the client's care providers.

When the TSI was implemented, the program's success was documented within several areas of intervention, among which, reducing challenging behaviors [106], enhancing motor and functional advancements [130], and improving the interaction of clients with family members [131].

The use of a MSE with individuals with IDD under the TSI method, enables an individually tailored intervention, with the therapists in charge of adapting the therapeutic program to each client beforehand while adapting each therapy session to the needs, demands, mood, and behavior of each client on a daily and even hourly basis. At the same time, the TSI method enables the collection of data presenting the gradual change of the service recipient.

5. Conclusion

Individuals with IDD are entitled to healthcare just as any other individual. However, despite their rights and although they are diagnosed with many more medical conditions necessitating proper health services and habilitation, they remain a marginal group of society that rarely receives the amount and quality of support they deserve. The current chapter was written to present the reader with up-to-date intervention methods to advance the opportunities for this group of clients.

Acknowledgements

The authors would like to thank the thousands of individuals with IDD who participated in our clinical work and research projects. Their involvement and needs are the source for constructing new evaluation and therapeutic methods. We thank them for teaching us how to properly care for them and become better therapists and human beings.

Conflict of interest

The authors declare no conflict of interest.

Author details

Meir Lotan[1]* and Alberto Romano[2]

1 Ariel University, Ariel, Israel

2 IRCCS Fondazione Don Carlo Gnocchi, Milan, Italy

*Address all correspondence to: meirlo@ariel.il

References

[1] Kadri M, Shiri S. Literature Review of the Diagnosys of People with Intellectual and Developmental Disability: Definition, Diagnostic Peroceedings and Phsychological Assessment Tools, Processes and Tools for Diagnosing co-Morbidity. Jerusalem, IS: Israeli Ministry of Social Affairs; 2015

[2] Shalom G, Ben Simchon M, Goren H. People with intellectual and developmental disability. In: Israeli Ministry of Social Affairs, editor. Social Service Review. Jerusalem, IS: Israeli Ministry of Social Affairs; 2016. p. 375

[3] Icht M, Ben-David N, Mama Y. Using vocal production to improve long-term verbal memory in adults with intellectual disability. Behavior Modification [Internet]. 2021;**45**:715-739. DOI: 10.1177/0145445520906583

[4] American Psychiatric Association. Diagnostic and Statistical Manual of Mental Disorders [Internet]. 5th ed. Washington, DC: American Psychiatric Association; 2013. Available from: https://psychiatryonline.org/doi/book/10.1176/appi.books.9780890425596 [Accessed: February 15, 2019]

[5] Redley M. Ageing and increased longevity amongst people with intellectual disabilities: An editorial. Quality in Ageing and Older Adults [Internet]. 2019;**20**:157-161. DOI: 10.1108/QAOA-12-2019-066/full/html

[6] Schalock RL, Borthwick-Duffy SA, Bradley VJ, Buntinx WHE, Coulter DL, Craig EM, et al. Intellectual Disability: Definition, Classification, and Systems of Supports. Washington, DC: American Association on Intellectual and Developmental Disabilities; 2010

[7] Patel DR, Greydanus DE, Merrick J, Rubin IL. Introduction to intellectual and developmental disabilities. In: Rubin IL, Merrick J, Greydanus DE, Patel DR, editors. Health Care for People with Intellectual and Developmental Disabilities across the Lifespan [Internet]. Cham, CH: Springer International Publishing; 2016. pp. 5-12. DOI: 10.1007/978-3-319-18096-0_1

[8] Polloway EA, Bouck EC, Patton JR, Lubin J. Intellectual and developmental disabilities. In: Kauffman JM, Hallahan DP, Paige CP, editors. Handbook of Special Education. 2nd ed. New York, NY: Routledge; 2017. pp. 265-285

[9] Eunice Kennedy Shriver National Institute of Child Health and Human Development. What Causes Intellectual and Developmental Disabilities (IDDs). Rockville, MD: Eunice Kennedy Shriver National Institute of Child Health and Human Development; 2021

[10] Simeonsson RJ. ICF-CY: A universal tool for documentation of disability. Journal of Policy and Practice in Intellectual Disabilities [Internet]. 2009;**6**:70-72. DOI: 10.1111/j.1741-1130.2009.00215.x

[11] Arvio M, Sillanpää M. Prevalence, aetiology and comorbidity of severe and profound intellectual disability in Finland. Journal of Intellectual Disability Research [Internet]. 2003;**47**:108-112

[12] Lotan M, Yalon-Chamovitz S, Weiss PLT. Improving physical fitness of individuals with intellectual and developmental disability through a virtual reality intervention program. Research in Developmental Disabilities [Internet]. 2009;**30**:229-239

[13] Blickwedel J, Ali A, Hassiotis A. Epilepsy and challenging behaviour in adults with intellectual disability: A systematic review. Journal of Intellectual & Developmental Disability [Internet]. 2019;**44**:219-231

[14] Schoen SA, Miller LJ, Sullivan J. The development and psychometric properties of the sensory processing scale inventory: A report measure of sensory modulation. Journal of Intellectual & Developmental Disability [Internet]. 2017;**42**:12-21. DOI: 10.3109/13668250.2016.1195490

[15] Perkins EA, Moran JA. Aging adults with intellectual disabilities. JAMA [Internet]. 2010;**304**:91-92. Available from: http://www.ncbi.nlm.nih.gov/pubmed/20606156

[16] Matson JL, Neal D. Psychotropic medication use for challenging behaviors in persons with intellectual disabilities: An overview. Research in Developmental Disabilities [Internet]. 2009;**30**:572-586. Available from: http://www.ncbi.nlm.nih.gov/pubmed/18845418

[17] Lin JD, Wu JL, Lee PN. Utilization of inpatient care and its determinants among persons with intellectual disabilities in day care centres in Taiwan. Journal of Intellectual Disability Research [Internet]. 2004;**48**:655-662. DOI: 10.1111/j.1365-2788.2003.00572.x

[18] Doran CM, Einfeld SL, Madden RH, Otim M, Horstead SK, Ellis LA, et al. How much does intellectual disability really cost? First estimates for Australia. Journal of Intellectual & Developmental Disability [Internet]. 2012;**37**:42-49. Available from: http://www.ncbi.nlm.nih.gov/pubmed/22339044

[19] Lotan M. Quality physical intervention activity for persons with down syndrome. The Scientific World Journal. 2007;**7**:7-19

[20] McCallion P, Ferretti LA, Beange H, McCarron M. Epidemiological issues in intellectual disability and aging research. In: Physical Health of Adults with Intellectual and Developmental Disabilities [Internet]. Cham: Springer International Publishing; 2019. pp. 9-26. DOI: 10.1007/978-3-319-90083-4_2

[21] Manduchi B, Fainman GM, Walshe M. Interventions for feeding and swallowing disorders in adults with intellectual disability: A systematic review of the evidence. Dysphagia [Internet]. 2020;**35**:207-219. Available from: http://www.ncbi.nlm.nih.gov/pubmed/31372756

[22] Beange H, Lennox N, Parmenter TR. Health targets for people with an intellectual disability. Journal of Intellectual & Developmental Disability [Internet]. 1999;**24**:283-297. Available from: https://www.tandfonline.com/doi/full/10.1080/13668259900034051

[23] Sinai A, Werner S, Stawski M. Assessing the need for a specialist service for people with intellectual disabilities and mental health problems living in Israel: A qualitative study. Frontiers in Pediatrics [Internet]. 2013;**1**:75970. DOI: 10.3389/fped.2013.00049/abstract

[24] Haveman M, Heller T, Lee L, Maaskant M, Shooshtari S, Strydom A. Major health risks in aging persons with intellectual disabilities: An overview of recent studies. Journal of Policy and Practice in Intellectual Disabilities [Internet]. 2010;**7**:59-69. DOI: 10.1111/j.1741-1130.2010.00248.x

[25] Bull FC, Al-Ansari SS, Biddle S, Borodulin K, Buman MP, Cardon G, et al. World Health Organization 2020 guidelines on physical activity and sedentary behaviour. British Journal of Sports Medicine [Internet]. 2020;**54**:1451-1462. Available

from: https://bjsm.bmj.com/content/54/24/1451

[26] World Health Organization. Global Recommendations on Physical Activity for Health. Geneva, CH: WHO Press; 2010

[27] Temple VA, Frey GC, Stanish HI. Physical activity of adults with mental retardation: Review and research needs [internet]. American Journal of Health Promotion. 2006;**21**:2-12. DOI: 101177/089011710602100103

[28] Lotan M, Isakov E, Kessel S, Merrick J. Physical fitness and functional ability of children with intellectual disability: Effects of a short-term daily treadmill intervention. The Scientific World Journal. 2004;**4**:449-457

[29] Grondhuis SN, Aman MG. Overweight and obesity in youth with developmental disabilities: A call to action. Journal of Intellectual Disability Research [Internet]. 2014;**58**:787-799. DOI: 10.1111/jir.12090

[30] Kapsal NJ, Dicke T, Morin AJS, Vasconcellos D, Maïano C, Lee J, et al. Effects of physical activity on the physical and psychosocial health of youth with intellectual disabilities: A systematic review and meta-analysis. Journal of Physical Activity and Health [Internet]. 2019;**16**:1187-1195. Available from: https://journals.humankinetics.com/view/journals/jpah/16/12/article-p1187.xml

[31] Jeng SC, Chang CW, Liu WY, Hou YJ, Lin YH. Exercise training on skill-related physical fitness in adolescents with intellectual disability: A systematic review and meta-analysis. Disability and Health Journal. 2017;**10**(2):198-206

[32] Shin IS, Park EY. Meta-analysis of the effect of exercise programs for individuals with intellectual disabilities. Research in Developmental Disabilities. 2012;**33**(6):1937-1947

[33] St. John L, Borschneck G, Cairney J. A systematic review and meta-analysis examining the effect of exercise on individuals with intellectual disability. American Journal on Intellectual and Developmental Disabilities [Internet]. 2020;**125**:274-286. DOI: 10.1352/1944-7558-125.4.274

[34] Maïano C, Hue O, Morin AJS, Lepage G, Tracey D, Moullec G. Exercise interventions to improve balance for young people with intellectual disabilities: A systematic review and meta-analysis. Developmental Medicine and Child Neurology. 2019;**61**(4):406-418

[35] Obrusnikova I, Firkin CJ, Farquhar WB. A systematic review and meta-analysis of the effects of aerobic exercise interventions on cardiorespiratory fitness in adults with intellectual disability. Disability and Health Journal. 2022;**15**(1):101185

[36] Harris L, Hankey C, Murray H, Melville C. The effects of physical activity interventions on preventing weight gain and the effects on body composition in young adults with intellectual disabilities: Systematic review and meta-analysis of randomized controlled trials. Clinical Obesity. 2015;**5**(4):198-210

[37] Yang W, Liang X, Sit CHP. Physical activity and mental health in children and adolescents with intellectual disabilities: A meta-analysis using the RE-AIM framework. International Journal of Behavioral Nutrition and Physical Activity. 2022;**19**(1):80

[38] Lynch L, McCarron M, McCallion P, Burke E. Sedentary behaviour levels in adults with an intellectual disability: A

systematic review and meta-analysis. HRB Open Research [Internet]. 2021;4:69. Available from: /pmc/articles/PMC9020532/

[39] Boman C, Bernhardsson S. Exploring needs, barriers, and facilitators for promoting physical activity for children with intellectual developmental disorders: A qualitative focus group study. Journal of Intellectual Disabilities. 2023;**27**:5-23

[40] Frey GC, Stanish HI, Temple VA. Physical activity of youth with intellectual disability: Review and research agenda. Adapted Physical Activity Quarterly. 2008;**25**:95-117

[41] McGarty AM, Downs SJ, Melville CA, Harris L. A systematic review and meta-analysis of interventions to increase physical activity in children and adolescents with intellectual disabilities. Journal of Intellectual Disability Research. 2018;**62**:312-329

[42] Jacinto M, Vitorino AS, Palmeira D, Antunes R, Ferreira JP, Bento T, et al. Perceived barriers of physical activity participation in individuals with intellectual disability—A systematic review. Healthcare (Switzerland). 2021;**9**(11):1521

[43] Pestana MB, Barbieri FA, Vitório R, Figueiredo GA, Mauerberg-deCastro E. Effects of physical exercise for adults with intellectual disabilities: A systematic review. Journal of Physical Education (Maringa). 2018;**41**(26):3118-3140

[44] Dixon-Ibarra A, Driver S, Vanderbom K, Humphries K. Understanding physical activity in the group home setting: A qualitative inquiry. Disability and Rehabilitation. 2017;**39**:653-662

[45] Romano A, Ippolito E, Favetta M, Lotan M, Moran DS. Individualized remotely supervised motor activity programs promote rehabilitation goal achievement, motor functioning, and physical activity of people with Rett syndrome—A single-cohort study. International Journal of Environmental Research and Public Health [Internet]. 2022;**20**:659. Available from: https://www.mdpi.com/1660-4601/20/1/659

[46] Bossink LWM, van der Putten AA, Vlaskamp C. Understanding low levels of physical activity in people with intellectual disabilities: A systematic review to identify barriers and facilitators. Research in Developmental Disabilities. 2017;**68**:95-110

[47] Shields N, Synnot AJ, Barr M. Perceived barriers and facilitators to physical activity for children with disability: A systematic review. British Journal of Sports Medicine. 2012;**46**(14):989-997

[48] Aherne C, Coughlan B. A preliminary investigation of the suitability of aquatics for people with severe and profound intellectual disabilities. Journal of Intellectual Disabilities. 2017;**21**:118-133

[49] Temple VA, Frey GC, Stanish HI. Interventions to promote physical activity for adults with intellectual disabilities. Salud Pública de México. 2017;**59**:446-453

[50] Hassan NM, Landorf KB, Shields N, Munteanu SE. Effectiveness of interventions to increase physical activity in individuals with intellectual disabilities: A systematic review of randomised controlled trials. Journal of Intellectual Disability Research. 2019;**63**(2):168-191

[51] Mahy J, Shields N, Taylor NF, Dodd KJ. Identifying facilitators and barriers to physical activity for adults

with down syndrome. Journal of Intellectual Disability Research. 2010;**54**:795-805

[52] Van Biesen D, Van Damme T, Morgulec-Adamowicz N, Buchholz A, Anjum M, Healy S. A systematic review of digital interventions to promote physical activity in people with intellectual disabilities and/or autism. Adapted Physical Activity Quarterly. 2023:1-21. DOI: 10.1123/apaq.2023-0061

[53] Beange HP. Caring for a vulnerable population: Who will take responsibility for those getting a raw deal from the health care system? The Medical Journal of Australia. 1996;**164**:159-160

[54] Harris JC. Intellectual Disability: Understanding its Development, Causes, Classification, Evaluation, and Treatment. Developmental Perspectives in Psychiatry. New York, NY: Oxford University Press; 2006

[55] Olympics S. Changing Attitudes Changing the World: The Health and Health Care of People with Intellectual Disabilities. Washington, DC: Special Olympics; 2005

[56] Walsh PN, Kerr M, van Schrojenstein Lantman-de Valk HMJ. Health indicators for people with intellectual disabilities: A European perspective. European Journal of Public Health [Internet]. 2003;**13**:47-50. Available from: http://www.ncbi.nlm.nih.gov/pubmed/14533748

[57] Fisher K. Health disparities and mental retardation. Journal of Nursing Scholarship [Internet]. 2004;**36**:48-53. Available from: http://www.ncbi.nlm.nih.gov/pubmed/15098418

[58] Bernal J, Tuffrey-Wijne I. Telling the truth – or not: Disclosure and information for people with intellectual disabilities who have cancer. International Journal on Disability and Human Development [Internet]. 2008;7:365-370. DOI: 10.1515/IJDHD.2008.7.4.365/html

[59] Janicki MP, Dalton AJ, Henderson CM, Davidson PW. Mortality and morbidity among older adults with intellectual disability: Health services considerations. Disability and Rehabilitation [Internet]. 1999;**21**:284-294. Available from: http://www.ncbi.nlm.nih.gov/pubmed/10381241

[60] Ben-David N, Lotan M, Moran DS. Association of COVID-19-related restrictions with changes in functional skills of adults with intellectual disabilities in day programs of an Israeli non-profit organization. Research and Practice for Persons with Severe Disabilities [Internet]. 2023;**48**:79-91. DOI: 10.1177/15407969231173929

[61] Ben-David N, Lotan M, Moran DS. A new screening tool for rapid diagnosis of functional and environmental factors influencing adults with intellectual disabilities. Diagnostics [Internet]. 2022;**12**:2991. Available from: https://www.mdpi.com/2075-4418/12/12/2991

[62] Ben-David N, Lotan M, Moran DS. Development and validation of a functional screening tool for adults with intellectual disabilities. Journal of Applied Research in Intellectual Disabilities [Internet]. 2022;**35**:1281-1296. DOI: 10.1111/jar.13004

[63] Heller T, Ying Gs G, Rimmer JH, Marks BA. Determinants of exercise in adults with cerebral palsy. Public Health Nursing [Internet]. 2002;**19**:223-231. Available from: http://www.ncbi.nlm.nih.gov/pubmed/11967109

[64] Tao D, Gao Y, Cole A, Baker JS, Gu Y, Supriya R, et al. The physiological and psychological benefits of dance and

its effects on children and adolescents: A systematic review. Frontiers in Physiology [Internet]. 2022;**13**:925958. DOI: 10.3389/fphys.2022.925958/full

[65] World Health Organization. International Classification of Functioning, Disability and Health : ICF. [Internet]. Geneva, CH: World Health Organization; 2001. Available from: https://books.google.it/books?hl=it&lr=&id=lMZPmEJrJ3sC&oi=fnd&pg=PA1&dq=World+Health+Organization.+International+Classification+of+Functioning,+Disability+and+Health.+Geneva:+World+Health+Organization,+2001.&ots=PGmESDf1Cc&sig=TljMRUIIj3T0qXOuIfYtfskvreo [Accessed: June 8, 2019]

[66] United Nations. Convention on the rights of persons with disabilities [internet]. In: Sixty-First Session of the General Assembly by Resolution A/RES/61/106. New York, NY: United Nations; 2006. Available from: https://www.ohchr.org/en/instruments-mechanisms/instruments/convention-rights-persons-disabilities [Accessed: January 8, 2024]

[67] Turner LA, Johnson B. A model of mastery motivation for at-risk preschoolers. Journal of Educational Psychology [Internet]. 2003;**95**:495-505. DOI: 10.1037/0022-0663.95.3.495

[68] Gilmore L, Cuskelly M. A longitudinal study of motivation and competence in children with down syndrome: Early childhood to early adolescence. Journal of Intellectual Disability Research [Internet]. 2009;**53**:484-492. Available from: http://www.ncbi.nlm.nih.gov/pubmed/19302472

[69] Deci EL. Promoting intrinsic motivation and self-determination in people with mental retardation. International Review of Research in Mental Retardation [Internet]. 2004;**28**:1-29. Available from: https://linkinghub.elsevier.com/retrieve/pii/S0074775004280016 [Accessed: January 8, 2024]

[70] Greenspan S. Functional concepts in mental retardation: Finding the natural essence of an artificial category. Exceptionality [Internet]. 2006;**14**:205-224. DOI: 10.1207/s15327035ex1404_3

[71] Chien C-W, Rodger S, Copley J. Differences in patterns of physical participation in recreational activities between children with and without intellectual and developmental disability. Research in Developmental Disabilities [Internet]. 2017;**67**:9-18. Available from: https://linkinghub.elsevier.com/retrieve/pii/S0891422217301348

[72] Hutzler Y, Korsensky O. Motivational correlates of physical activity in persons with an intellectual disability: A systematic literature review. Journal of Intellectual Disability Research [Internet]. 2010;**54**:767-786. Available from: http://www.ncbi.nlm.nih.gov/pubmed/20712695

[73] Caprì T, Nucita A, Iannizzotto G, Stasolla F, Romano A, Semino M, et al. Telerehabilitation for improving adaptive skills of children and young adults with multiple disabilities: A systematic review. Review Journal of Autism and Developmental Disorders. 2021;**8**:244-252

[74] World Health Organization. The World Bank. World Report on Disability. Geneva, CH: World Health Organization; 2011

[75] Ptomey LT, Szabo AN, Willis EA, Greene JL, Danon JC, Washburn RA, et al. Remote exercise for adults with down syndrome. Translational Journal of

the American College of Sports Medicine [Internet]. 2018;3:60. Available from: /pmc/articles/PMC6005664/

[76] Lotan M, Ippolito E, Favetta M, Romano A. Skype supervised, individualized, home-based rehabilitation programs for individuals with Rett syndrome and their families – parental satisfaction and point of view. Frontiers in Psychology [Internet]. 2021;**12**:3995. DOI: 10.3389/fpsyg.2021.720927/full

[77] Romano A, Di Rosa G, Tisano A, Fabio RA, Lotan M. Effects of a remotely supervised motor rehabilitation program for individuals with Rett syndrome at home. Disability and Rehabilitation [Internet]. 2021;**44**:1-11. DOI: 10.1080/09638288.2021.1949398

[78] Rimmer JH, Wang E, Pellegrini CA, Lullo C, Gerber BS. Telehealth weight management intervention for adults with physical disabilities: A randomized controlled trial. American Journal of Physical Medicine & Rehabilitation [Internet]. 2013;**92**:1084-1094. Available from: http://journals.lww.com/00002060-201312000-00006

[79] Vismara LA, McCormick C, Young GS, Nadhan A, Monlux K. Preliminary findings of a telehealth approach to parent training in autism. Journal of Autism and Developmental Disorders. 2013;**43**:2953-2969

[80] Shahrbanian S, Kateb MY, Doyle-Baker PK, Hassani F. Physical activity for children with autism spectrum disorder during COVID-19 pandemic. International Journal of Developmental Disabilities [Internet]. 2023;69:467. Available from: /pmc/articles/PMC10281427/

[81] Simacek J, Dimian AF, McComas JJ. Communication intervention for young children with severe neurodevelopmental disabilities via telehealth. Journal of Autism and Developmental Disorders. 2017;**47**:744-767

[82] Baharav E, Reiser C. Using telepractice in parent training in early autism. Telemedicine and e-Health [Internet]. 2010;**16**:727-731. Available from: https://www.liebertpub.com/doi/10.1089/tmj.2010.0029

[83] Barlow IG, Liu L, Sekulic A. Wheelchair seating assessment and intervention: A comparison between telerehabilitation and face-to-face service. International Journal of Telerehabilitation. 2009;**1**:17

[84] Schein RM, Schmeler MR, Holm MB, Pramuka M, Saptono A, Brienza DM. Telerehabilitation assessment using the functioning everyday with a wheelchair-capacity instrument. Journal of Rehabilitation Research and Development. 2011;**48**:115-124

[85] Hoffmann T, Russell T. Pre-admission orthopaedic occupational therapy home visits conducted using the internet. Journal of Telemedicine and Telecare. 2008;**14**:83-87

[86] Hoffmann T, Russell T, Thompson L, Vincent A, Nelson M. Using the internet to assess activities of daily living and hand function in people with Parkinson's disease. NeuroRehabilitation. 2008;**23**:253-261

[87] Cason J, Cohn ER. Telepractice: An overview and best practices. Perspectives of Augmentative and Alternative Communication. 2014;**23**:4-17

[88] Kelso GL, Fiechtl BJ, Olsen ST, Rule S. The feasibility of virtual home visits to provide early intervention: A pilot study. Infants & Young Children [Internet]. 2009;**22**:332-340. Available

from: https://journals.lww.com/iycjournal/fulltext/2009/10000/the_feasibility_of_virtual_home_visits_to_provide.9.aspx

[89] Cason J, Behl D, Ringwalt S. Overview of states' use of telehealth for the delivery of early intervention (IDEA part C) services. International Journal of Telerehabilitation. 2012;**4**:39

[90] Camden C, Pratte G, Fallon F, Couture M, Berbari J, Tousignant M. Diversity of practices in telerehabilitation for children with disabilities and effective intervention characteristics: Results from a systematic review. Disability and Rehabilitation [Internet]. 2020;**42**:3424-3436. DOI: 10.1080/09638288.2019.1595750

[91] Romano A, Ippolito E, Risoli C, Malerba E, Favetta M, Sancesario A, et al. Intensive postural and motor activity program reduces scoliosis progression in people with Rett syndrome. Journal of Clinical Medicine [Internet]. 2022;**11**:559. Available from: https://www.mdpi.com/2077-0383/11/3/559

[92] Lotan M, Stahlhut M, Romano A, Downs J, Elefant C. Family-centered telehealth supporting motor skills and activity in individuals with Rett syndrome. In: Stasolla F, editor. Assistive Technologies for Assessment and Recovery of Neurological Impairments [Internet]. Hershey, PA: IGI Global; 2022. pp. 147-171. DOI: 10.4018/978-1-7998-7430-0.ch008

[93] Standen PJ, Brown DJ, Cromby JJ. The effective use of virtual environments in the education and rehabilitation of students with intellectual disabilities. British Journal of Educational Technology [Internet]. 2001;**32**:289-299. DOI: 10.1111/1467-8535.00199

[94] Oppewal A, Hilgenkamp TIM, Schäfer Elinder L, Freiberger E, Rintala P, Guerra-Balic M, et al. Correlates of sedentary behaviour in adults with intellectual disabilities-a systematic review. International Journal of Environmental Research and Public Health [Internet]. 2018;**15**:2274. Available from: http://www.ncbi.nlm.nih.gov/pubmed/30336554

[95] Rizzo A, "Skip", Kim GJ. A SWOT analysis of the field of virtual reality rehabilitation and therapy. Presence: Teleoperators and Virtual Environments [Internet]. 2005;**14**:119-146. Available from: https://direct.mit.edu/pvar/article/14/2/119-146/18546

[96] Weiss PL, Kizony R, Feintuch U, Katz N. Virtual reality in neurorehabilitation. In: Textbook of Neural Repair and Rehabilitation [Internet]. Cambridge, UK: Cambridge University Press; 2006. pp. 182-197. Available from: https://www.cambridge.org/core/product/identifier/CBO9780511545078A028/type/book_part

[97] Eden S, Bezer M. Three-dimensions vs. two-dimensions intervention programs: The effect on the mediation level and behavioural aspects of children with intellectual disability. European Journal of Special Needs Education [Internet]. 2011;**26**:337-353. DOI: 10.1080/08856257.2011.593827

[98] Parsons S, Mitchell P. The potential of virtual reality in social skills training for people with autistic spectrum disorders. Journal of Intellectual Disability Research [Internet]. 2002;**46**:430-443. Available from: http://www.ncbi.nlm.nih.gov/pubmed/12031025

[99] Rheingold H. Virtual Reality: [The Revolutionary Technology of Computer-Generated Artificial Worlds and How it Promises to Transform Society]. New York: Simon & Schuster; 1992

[100] Tam S-F, Man DW-K, Chan Y-P, Sze P-C, Wong C-M. Evaluation of a computer-assisted, 2-D virtual reality system for training people with intellectual disabilities on how to shop. Rehabilitation Psychology [Internet]. 2005;**50**:285-291. DOI: 10.1037/0090-5550.50.3.285

[101] Tamar Weiss PL, Bialik P, Kizony R. Virtual reality provides leisure time opportunities for young adults with physical and intellectual disabilities. Cyberpsychology, Behavior, and Social Networking [Internet]. 2003;**6**:335-342. DOI: 10.1089/109493103322011650

[102] Standen PJ, Brown DJ. Virtual reality in the rehabilitation of people with intellectual disabilities: Review. Cyberpsychology, Behavior, and Social Networking [Internet]. 2005;**8**:272-282. DOI: 10.1089/cpb.2005.8.272

[103] Lotan M, Yalon-Chamovitz S, Weiss PL, (Tamar). Training caregivers to provide virtual reality intervention for adults with severe intellectual and developmental disability. Journal of Physical Therapy Education [Internet]. 2011;**25**:15-19. Available from: http://journals.lww.com/00001416-201110000-00004

[104] Yalon-Chamovitz S, Weiss PL, (Tamar). Virtual reality as a leisure activity for young adults with physical and intellectual disabilities. Research in Developmental Disabilities. 2008;**29**:273-287

[105] Lotan M, Weiss L, P. Improving balance in adults with intellectual developmental disorder via virtual environments. Perceptual and Motor Skills [Internet]. 2021;**128**:2638-2653. Available from: http://www.ncbi.nlm.nih.gov/pubmed/34632865

[106] Mengue-Topio H, Courbois Y, Farran EK, Sockeel P. Route learning and shortcut performance in adults with intellectual disability: A study with virtual environments. Research in Developmental Disabilities [Internet]. 2011;**32**:345-352. Available from: https://linkinghub.elsevier.com/retrieve/pii/S0891422210002520

[107] Wright T, Wolery M. The effects of instructional interventions related to street crossing and individuals with disabilities. Research in Developmental Disabilities [Internet]. 2011;**32**:1455-1463. Available from: https://linkinghub.elsevier.com/retrieve/pii/S0891422211001387

[108] Cooke P, Laczny A, Brown DJ, Francik J. The virtual courtroom: A view of justice. Project to prepare witnesses or victims with learning disabilities to give evidence. Disability and Rehabilitation [Internet]. 2002;**24**:634-642. DOI: 10.1080/09638280110111414

[109] Tarnanas I, Manos GC. Using virtual reality to teach special populations how to cope in crisis: The case of a virtual earthquake. Studies in Health Technology and Informatics [Internet]. 2001;**81**:495-501. DOI: 10.3233/978-1-60750-925-7-495

[110] Wuang Y-P, Chiang C-S, Su C-Y, Wang C-C. Effectiveness of virtual reality using Wii gaming technology in children with down syndrome. Research in Developmental Disabilities [Internet]. 2011;**32**:312-321. Available from: http://www.ncbi.nlm.nih.gov/pubmed/21071171

[111] Passig D. Improving the sequential time perception of teenagers with mild to moderate mental retardation with 3D immersive virtual reality (IVR). Journal of Educational Computing Research [Internet]. 2009;**40**:263-280. DOI: 10.2190/EC.40.3.a

[112] Akhutina T, Foreman N, Krichevets A, Matikka L, Narhi V,

Pylaeva N, et al. Improving spatial functioning in children with cerebral palsy using computerized and traditional game tasks. Disability and Rehabilitation [Internet]. 2003;**25**:1361-1371. DOI: 10.1080/09638280310001616358

[113] Standen P, Cromby J, Brown D. Playing for real. Journal of Mental Health Care. 1998;**1**:412-415

[114] Walker HM, Sylwester R. Reducing students' refusal and resistance. Teaching exceptional children [Internet]. 1998;**30**:52-58. DOI: 10.1177/004005999803000610

[115] Booth V, Masud T, Connell L, Bath-Hextall F. The effectiveness of virtual reality interventions in improving balance in adults with impaired balance compared with standard or no treatment: A systematic review and meta-analysis. Clinical Rehabilitation [Internet]. 2014;**28**:419-431. Available from: http://www.ncbi.nlm.nih.gov/pubmed/24188913

[116] Da Cunha RD, Neiva FW, Silva RL DDS. Virtual reality as a support tool for the treatment of people with intellectual and multiple disabilities: A systematic literature review. Revista de Informática Teórica e Aplicada [Internet]. 2018;**25**:67. Available from: http://seer.ufrgs.br/index.php/rita/article/view/RITA_VOL25_NR1_67

[117] McMahon AK, McMahon DD. Exercise technology interventions and individuals with IDD. Division on Autism and Developmental Disabilities Online Journal. 2016;**3**:42-53

[118] Ayres AJ, Robbins J. Sensory Integration and the Child: Understanding Hidden Sensory Challenges. Los Angeles, CA: Western Psychological Services; 2005

[119] Longhorn F. Planning a Multisensory Massage Programme for Very Special People. Austin, TX: Catalyst Education Resources, Ltd; 1993

[120] Hulsegge J, Verheul A. Snoezelen: Another World. Chesterfield, UK: Rompa; 1987

[121] Shapiro M, Snoezeling BS. Controlled Multi-Sensory Stimulation. A Handbook for Practitioners. Ra'anana, IL: Beit Issie Shapiro; 2002

[122] Kerr AM, Belichenko P, Woodcock T, Woodcock M. Mind and brain in Rett disorder. Brain & Development. 2001;**23**:S44-S49

[123] Kerr A. Annotation: Rett syndrome: Recent progress and implications for research and clinical practice. Journal of Child Psychology and Psychiatry [Internet]. 2002;**43**:277-287. DOI: 10.1111/1469-7610.00021

[124] Elefant C. Music, Choice Making and Communication in Rett Syndrome. Ostersund, SE: A lecture presented at the International Course on Rett Syndrome; 2003

[125] Grocke D, Wigram T. Receptive Methods in Music Therapy: Techniques and Clinical Applications for Music Therapy Clinicians, Educators and Students. Jessica Kingsley Publishers; 2007

[126] Kerr AM. How Can we Help the Youngest Ones with Rett Disorder? Northampton, UK: A lecture presented at the annual Riding for the Disabled Association UK family weekend; 2002

[127] Kerr AM. Infant development in Rett syndrome. In: A Lecture Presented at the International Course on Rett Syndrome. Ostersund, SE; 2003

[128] Verheul A. Snoezelen. Hrezelia, IL: International Snoezelen Conference; 2004

[129] Lotan M, Gold C, Yalon-Chamovitz S. Reducing challenging behavior through structured therapeutic intervention in the controlled multi-sensory environment (Snoezelen). Ten case studies. International Journal on Disability and Human Development [Internet]. 2009;**8**:377-392. DOI: 10.1515/IJDHD.2009.8.4.377/html

[130] Lotan M, Burshtein S. Physical Therapy Intervention for Senior Citizens with Cognitive Impairment. Chicago, IL, US: American Association on Mental Retardation (AAMR) Annual Meeting; 2003

[131] Nasser K, Cahana C, Kandel I, Kessel S, Merrick J. Snoezelen: Children with intellectual disability and working with the whole family. The Scientific World Journal [Internet]. 2004;**4**:500-506. Available from: https://www.hindawi.com/journals/tswj/2004/939745/